MEDITERRANEAN DIET FOR BEGINNERS

A Quick Start Guide to Heart-Healthy Eating, Supercharged Weight Loss, and Unstoppable Energy

Including 30 MINUTE Mediterranean Diet Recipes and a 7-Day Meal Plan

Gina Crawford

2016 – NEW Extended edition with bonus information and recipes

Copyright © 2015 by Gina Crawford

Evita Publishing, PO Box 306, Station A, Vancouver Island, BC V9W 5B1 Canada

IMPORTANT

The information in this book reflects the author's research, experiences, and opinions and is not intended to replace medical advice.

Before beginning this or any nutritional or exercise regimen, consult your physician to be sure it is appropriate for you. Ask for a physical stress test.

Table of Contents

Introduction

Welcome to the all new 2016 extended edition of the *Mediterranean Diet for Beginners!*

The Mayo Clinic termed the Mediterranean diet a heart-healthy diet.....and rightly so! Eating the Mediterranean way will help you prevent heart disease, diabetes, cancer, and many other life-threatening diseases. It will enhance the quality of your life, help you lose weight, and increase your energy.

As a plant-based, whole foods diet, the traditional Mediterranean diet has great respect for nature and life itself. It recognizes the importance of eating foods in their most natural state and it reminds us to slow down and savor both food and life on a daily basis.

It also recognizes the importance of balance and suggests eating a wide variety of foods daily in order to get the vitamins, minerals and phytonutrients that different plant foods offer.

When you eat the Mediterranean way you nourish your body in a way that allows it to function at its best.

In this book, I have explained the traditional Mediterranean diet in a straight forward, to the point way that will allow you to learn everything you need to know about how to successfully apply the diet to your life in a short amount of time.

I truly believe in the traditional Mediterranean diet and know from experience that it will help you lose weight, improve your health, and make you more energetic than ever! My hope is that you will use the information in this book to live a long and healthy life. Enjoy!

A Note About Measurements in This Book

For my UK friends: In order to get the most accurate measurements for each recipe in this book, I highly recommend purchasing a set of North American measuring cups (a liquid measure and a dry measure). You can purchase a set of each online. This will make cooking these delicious recipes a breeze!

Chapter 1

What is the Mediterranean Diet?

"The doctor of the future will no longer treat the human frame with drugs, but rather will cure and prevent disease with nutrition."
Thomas Edison

The Mediterranean diet isn't actually a diet. Yes, it can help you lose weight and maintain or improve your health, but it's really more of a lifestyle. It's a way of eating that can nurture your health for life.

The Mediterranean diet, universally known as the gold standard way of eating, is based on the traditional dietary patterns of the countries that border the Mediterranean Sea like Greece, Spain, Israel, Italy, and France. It gained widespread popularity in the west during the 1990's and since then has become the world's most respected diet, particularly for its heart-health and longevity benefits.

There are 21 countries that border the Mediterranean Sea and though their diets, culture, agriculture, ethnic background, and economy vary there are common dietary patterns that they share. These common patterns have become characteristic of what we call the Mediterranean diet.

The most authentic version of the Mediterranean diet is based on the dietary patterns of the people of Crete (the largest Greek island) during the 1950's and 1960's. Their eating habits and lifestyle are now referred to as the traditional Mediterranean diet.

The traditional Mediterranean diet encompasses all of the health benefits that are scientifically documented. Unfortunately, a more modern version of the Mediterranean diet has emerged over the years that has compromised the foundational characteristics of the diet.

In place of organic plant foods, seafood, nuts, olive oil, herbs and spices, the Mediterranean diet of today has become synonymous with foods like pizza, spaghetti with meat sauce, lasagna, gyros, and bottomless bowls of pasta. Large family gatherings where everyone is enjoying limitless amounts of food and red wine with the motto eat, drink and be merry is what people envision when they think of the Mediterranean diet.

The problem with this view is that it propagates excess and imbalance. Yes, the Mediterranean diet incorporates foods like pizza and spaghetti, and there is no question that gatherings that involve food are important, but the modern view of this is excessive. Pizzas loaded with cheese, spaghetti sauce packed with meat, and eating as much bread and pasta as you want are all embellishments that have only served to increase calories, unhealthy fats, obesity, heart disease, diabetes, and other health problems.

In order to understand and reap the health benefits from the traditional version of the Mediterranean diet that scientific studies are based on it's important to first look at the foundational characteristics that make up the traditional Mediterranean diet.

Characteristics of the traditional Mediterranean diet according to researchers

A high consumption of food from plant sources is recommended. Plant foods are the foundation of the diet.

Each meal includes fruits, vegetables, and grains. Most grains like oats, rice, wheat, barley, corn, and rye are consumed whole with minimal processing. Fresh fruit is a typical dessert.

Nuts, seeds, legumes, and beans are rich in good fat and protein. They are consumed often and are considered an important part of the diet.

Emphasis is on seasonal, locally grown, antioxidant and micronutrient rich fresh produce that is minimally processed.

Olives and olive oil are the primary source of monounsaturated fat replacing other oils and fats, including margarine and butter.

Fish and shellfish are an important source of omega-3 fatty acids on the diet.

Herbs and spices are used to enhance the flavor of food. They provide antioxidants and are often used in place of salt.

Red wine is consumed in moderation and is typically served with a meal.

Dairy is consumed in moderation.

Eggs are consumed in moderation.

Low consumption of red meat is recommended with moderate amounts of poultry.

Sweets are savored and appreciated in small amounts.

Portion size is considered at each meal.

Adequate daily water intake is important.

Food is considered a pleasure that involves sharing meals and drinks with family and friends.

Daily exercise is a way of life. It can range from moderate to strenuous.

Slowing down, savoring food, and enjoying life are important aspects of the diet.

Why choose the Mediterranean diet?

The Mediterranean diet is the most scientifically documented diet in the world.

It is a complete and balanced diet that provides the body with all the nutrients it needs to function at its best.

Its emphasis on plant foods provides the body with phytochemicals and HDL boosting monounsaturated fats that are an essential part of a healthy diet.

The Mediterranean diet uses common foods that are readily available. This makes it easy for anyone to implement.

Chapter 2

A Brief History of the Mediterranean Diet

The origins of the Mediterranean diet date back to the Middle Ages when the upper class ancient Romans (modeling Greek tradition) would regularly consume wine, bread, olive oil, vegetables, fruit, sheep cheese, an abundance of fish, various seafood, and little red meat.

The health benefits of the Mediterranean diet were discovered by American scientist Ancel Benjamin Keys who avidly studied the influence of diet on health. His studies on the Mediterranean diet were the first to reveal a correlation between cardiovascular disease and diet.

How the benefits of the Mediterranean diet were discovered

Ancel Keys, after which K-rations were named in 1939, became interested in studying the effects of semistarvation on the human body during World War II when millions of people suffered from a lack of food due to the disruption of food supplies.

In 1950 he published his research on identifying the effects of semistarvation and restoring the body back to health in a 1300+ page book called

The Biology of Human Starvation that has since become a highly respected and referenced classic work in the field of human starvation.

Keys work on starvation allowed him to have access to data on health and disease in post-war Europe. As he studied the data, he was intrigued to find a correlation between a lower rate of heart attacks in countries that did not have their usual access to high-fat, high-calorie foods during the war. When their usual high-fat, high-calorie foods were restored after the war, Keys noticed a rise in the rate of heart attacks. He was also perplexed by a recent rise in the amount of heart attacks in wealthy American middle-aged businessmen.

This led him to conduct a study on 283 businessman and professionals in the Minnesota area that were between the ages of 45 and 55. His goal was to see if there was a correlation between diet, saturated fat intake, blood cholesterol levels, and clotting in coronary arteries. Keys study ran for 40 years. From this study, he discovered that the major cause of death was heart disease due to high cholesterol.

In 1951 Keys traveled to Oxford on a one year sabbatical. While there, an Italian colleague proudly told him that there was almost no heart disease at all in Italy. Keys of course found this hard to believe. Luckily, Keys decided to investigate this himself by setting up a lab in Naples. Eventually, he was able to verify that people in Naples did in fact have a lower rate of heart disease along with surprisingly low serum cholesterol levels.

Keys continued this research into other European as well as African countries. Soon he started seeing a pattern. He noticed that diets high in saturated fats caused serum cholesterol levels to rise. This was the main cause of coronary heart disease.

In 1955, at a time when suspecting diet as a major cause of heart disease was controversial, Keys shared his theory for the first time with the World Health Organization. His theory was met with skepticism yet Keys walked away more determined than ever to prove that his theory was correct.

The Seven Countries Study

Between 1955-1958 Keys initiated, organized and executed the world's first multi-country epidemiological longitudinal study called the Seven Countries Study. He organized teams of scientists and clinicians that would collectively work to answer their questions about heart and vascular disease among countries that had varied traditional eating habits and lifestyles.

The hypothesis was that the prevalence of coronary heart disease in individuals and populations would vary depending on the physical characteristics, lifestyle, and diet (particularly the intake of saturated fat and the level of serum cholesterol) of the people in each culture.

In order to conduct the study, participants had to be found, countries had to be selected, and testing techniques had to be developed. Researchers were required to do fieldwork which involved transporting awkwardly large medical equipment like electrocardiograph machines (that were much more primitive back then) to rural populations.

The seven countries that were specifically selected for the study were the United States, Italy, Japan, Greece, Finland, the Netherlands, and Yugoslavia. The study formally got underway in September 1958 and continued through to the early 1970's.

Researchers in each of the seven countries compiled data on over 12,000 healthy, middle-aged men between the ages of 40-59. As the data was collected it was sent back to Keys laboratory at the University of Minnesota. The database grew and cultural differences were translated into equations that could predict heart disease. Follow-up visits were conducted every five years after the initial visit.

The Seven Countries Study found that the lowest rates of heart attack occurred in Crete followed by Japan. The highest rates of heart attack occurred in East Finland.

In comparing Crete and East Finland, the heart attack rate in East Finland was extremely higher than Crete. Over a 10-year period 3.2% of the participants experienced a heart attack whereas in Crete the rate was only 0.1%.

During the study researchers also measured variables like physical activity, weight, blood cholesterol, resting heart rate, lung capacity, blood pressure, and smoking, and determined which ones could be correlated to heart attack rates.

Overall, the Seven Countries Study showed that the greatest risk factors for coronary heart disease were serum cholesterol, blood pressure, diabetes, and smoking.

The strongest lifestyle indicator of heart disease was saturated fat intake and the strongest physiological indicator of heart disease was blood cholesterol. The second strongest physiological indicator of heart disease was blood pressure.

Due to Keys research we know that blood pressure and blood cholesterol account for 60% of the risk of heart disease.

Through the Seven Countries Study, Keys proved that saturated fat intake could successfully predict cholesterol level. The study also showed that people can prevent cardiovascular disease through diet and that lifestyle choices can largely influence health.

Ancel Keys and his Seven Countries Study colleagues not only recognized and promoted the eating habits that they discovered in Crete in the 1950's and 1960's but they adopted this way of eating themselves. Keys was the first medical scientist to recognize and understand the power and immense benefits of the Mediterranean diet.

Keys in fact, was so impressed with the Mediterranean style of eating that he, along with his wife, a biochemist, wrote two books on the topic, *Eat Well and Stay Well*, and *How to Eat Well and Stay Well the Mediterranean Way*.

Keys lived in Italy for several years practicing everything that he preached about the

Mediterranean diet. He continued to work until he was 97 years old and died in 2004 at the age of 100.

The Seven Countries Study continues to this day still finding correlations between health, diet, lifestyle, disease, aging, well-being, and longevity.

Scientific proof of the benefits of the Mediterranean diet

Today, there are thousands of scientific studies that prove the effectiveness of the Mediterranean diet. Over 400 studies are published yearly.

The Mediterranean diet has more scientific proof of its effectiveness than any other diet.

Keys studies started a flood of scientific research that looked at the correlation between chronic disease and dietary habits. Many clinical trials and studies have proven that the Mediterranean diet reduces the risk of metabolic syndrome and cardiovascular disease.

Documented scientific studies have also proven that following a Mediterranean diet reduces high cholesterol by increasing high density lipoprotein (HDL), lowers blood pressure, triglycerides, blood glucose levels, and abdominal circumference, prevents chronic diseases, promotes longevity, improves cognitive function, fights cancer, prevents diabetes, Alzheimer's and Parkinson's, promotes weight loss, improves eye and dental health, helps fight depression, improves rheumatoid arthritis and more.

New studies appear regularly in leading scientific journals supporting the health benefits of the Mediterranean diet.

Chapter 3

Eating the Mediterranean Way

Traditional Mediterranean cuisine includes foods that are rich in colors, flavors and aromas and that reflect the spirit, oneness and beauty of living in harmony with nature.

Each country in the Mediterranean grows its own food and harvests it. This allows people living in the Mediterranean region to buy food that has been grown within miles of where they are. The closer the food, the fresher and more nutrient-rich it is. This is a sharp contrast to American grocery store chains that import produce from countries that are thousands of miles away. How fresh or nutrient-rich can that be?

Eating foods in season is of prime importance in Mediterranean countries. Pomegranates, grapes, cherries, persimmons, wild mushrooms, zucchini, spinach, cantaloupe, tomatoes, and olives are among the luscious fruits and vegetables grown in either spring or summer in the Mediterranean region.

In the summer, outdoor markets are very common. Vendors sell locally or regionally grown whole living foods that would shame the American pale produce found in mega grocery store chains.

Fresh fruit is the most common dessert in Mediterranean countries and vegetables are incorporated into every meal.

For most Americans it is a chore to eat enough fruits and vegetables in a day but for people in Mediterranean countries it is just a way of life.

Though the countries bordering the Mediterranean Sea have their own unique customs and culinary characteristics they are unified by common ingredients, herbs, spices, cooking techniques, and eating traditions.

Bread, for example, has long been considered a staple. In the more rural areas of the Mediterranean a loaf of bread is typically heavy, dark and packed with whole grains. Grains are also largely consumed as rice and various forms of pasta.

Legumes are also a staple and a great source of protein.

A touch of cheese is a common addition to a meal and it is never served in excess or smothered over a main meal. Just enough to be savored is satisfactory.

Red wine is another common addition to a main meal. It is also served in modest amounts, never in excess.

Chapter 4

The Mediterranean Diet... More Than Just Food

The Mediterranean diet in its most holistic and authentic form includes more than just food. It is an approach to eating and to life that involves taking the time to enjoy both.

Life is to be loved and savored, and food is an outward expression of that love and joy. There is also an inherent respect for food and life in Mediterranean countries. Nourishing the body with clean, whole natural foods is a way of honoring and respecting life.

For the Mediterranean people food also encompasses cultural as well as ethical and historical values. In other words, food is considered a pleasure. This pleasure is all about sharing food, socializing and spending time with others.

In Mediterranean countries, sharing meals together has always meant serenity and contentment.

Preparing food for twelve is hardly different than preparing food for four. It is a common way to share the beauty of food and life together.

Food is also seen as an important societal act.

The Mediterranean culture is connected by way of the marketplace, street, church, pub, and the square where people meet for food and share their lives and thoughts with each other.

Eating together is a cheerful act that strengthens relationships, offers relaxation and release, lessens stress, and creates social harmony. The act of cooking a meal, then setting the table and serving food is a way of life that gives importance to people and pleases the senses with flavors, smells, colors, rhythms, and images that are imbued with the Mediterranean spirit.

In traditional Mediterranean culture, the family unit was strong and neighbors and friends supported each other whenever a need arose.

Strong family ties and friendships are another aspect of the Mediterranean diet that contribute to better health. Family support and all weather friends can help to reduce the risk of disease, make the immune system stronger, slow aging, and lengthen life.

Mediterranean people simply know how to slow down, enjoy life and enjoy food. North American's don't value this as they should. Fast-food restaurants, fast-paced lives and materialism have overrun this simple yet profound principle of healthy living.

In Italy, Greece, and other Mediterranean countries it is very common for shops to close in the afternoon and re-open after shopkeepers have had a chance to go home, eat lunch with their kids and rest for a while. They recognize the importance of slowing down and enjoying life rather than stressfully running through it.

This is a very key part of the Mediterranean diet because the stress we incur by living a frantic life can take just as much of a toll on our health as eating poorly. It's important to do both, eat well and enjoy life by slowing down.

Mediterranean people have mastered the art of enjoying and appreciating the gifts of nature, delighting in foods, enjoying the company of others, and enjoying life itself. This quality enhances their health, lengthens their life, and ultimately gives them a deeper and richer life experience.

Chapter 5

How to Adopt a Mediterranean Lifestyle Using the Mediterranean Diet Food Pyramid

The Mediterranean diet food pyramid suggests daily servings for each of the different food groups. It is set up to provide a general sense of the proportions and frequency of food group servings that make up the dietary pattern of Mediterranean style eating.

The pyramid intentionally does not specify recommended weights of foods or calories so no calorie counting is necessary on the diet. The pyramid is only meant to provide an overall look at healthy food choices and the relative proportions.

It teaches you to switch out bad fats for good fats, choose fish and poultry instead of red meat, use olive oil instead of butter or margarine, be creative in incorporating fruits and vegetables into your daily food plan, consume beans, nuts and seeds regularly, switch out salt for herbs and spices, and let plant foods be the foundation of your daily food choices.

Good health has been attributed to variation within the overall dietary pattern. The more variety you get within the specified relative allowances per category, the better!

The Mediterranean diet is balanced and does not cut out major food groups. Bread is something that is often looked at as taboo when it comes to dieting, but not with the Mediterranean diet!

What makes the Mediterranean diet so effective is the combination of foods in the pyramid. High fiber, good fat, and phytochemicals from plant foods provide a balanced, non-nutritionally deficient diet that promotes great health.

The pyramid recommends serving sizes for each category since portion control is an important part of the Mediterranean diet. Moderation is key.

How much you eat in total depends on your body's unique caloric needs. Special dietary requirements should be taken into consideration.

A dietician or health care provider can help you determine the nutrients you need as well as how many calories you should consume per day.

Components of the Mediterranean Diet Pyramid

Water

In addition to diligently adhering to the Mediterranean diet food groups and servings, it is also vital that you understand the importance of daily water consumption on the diet.

Water consumption is an extremely important part of any diet. While on the Mediterranean diet it is important to consume the amount of water that your body needs on a daily basis.

Water is necessary for almost every bodily function because it helps carry essential nutrients to all our cells. An average person can live up to forty-five days without food, but only three to five days without water.

There are many people suffering from dehydration on a regular basis because they don't consume enough fluids to keep their vital organs saturated with water.

The perils of dehydration

Approximately two-thirds of our body weight is water. The human body is made up of about 60% water. Our brain cells are made up of about 85% water, muscles are about 75% water, blood is about 82% water and our bones are about 25% water. The average-sized person requires 64-96 ounces of water every day in order to satisfy the body's need for it.

When your body becomes dehydrated it begins to ration its water supply. The body's first priority is to keep the vital organs hydrated, so it works overtime pulling water from other areas of the body in order to do this. The organs that the body considers vital are the heart, lungs, brain, liver, and kidneys. Other systems such as the skin, joints, and gastrointestinal tract are considered less important. That is why the negative symptoms of dehydration usually show up there first.

A lack of water also causes a loss of water volume in the cells which affects the body's effectiveness in delivering vital nutrients to cells, and excreting waste from cells. This causes constipation which can cause rectal diseases like hemorrhoids, diverticulitis, chronic constipation, and spastic colon.

A shortage of water can also contribute to high blood pressure, asthma, allergies, heart disease, ulcers, arthritis, back and neck pain, headaches, memory loss, kidney stones, hernias, and high cholesterol.

Remember: Thirst is not the first sign of dehydration. By the time you get thirsty or experience a dry mouth your cells are already desperately craving water.

How much water do you need?

US News and World Report ran an article in 2013 entitled *The Truth About How Much Water You Should Really Drink.* This article stated that in order to determine how much water your body needs you must first calculate how much water your body requires at rest. "At rest" would be considered non-vigorous activities like reading or working at a desk.

In order to calculate this, divide your body weight in half. For example, if you weigh 150 pounds then your body requires 75 ounces of water every day. If you weigh 140 pounds then your body requires 70 ounces of water every day.

If you work out in a day you will need to increase that number because you will be losing water through sweat.

There are also special cases when it comes to daily recommended water intake. For example those who suffer from kidney stones or chronic urinary tract infections will have to drink more water.

The elderly may need to adjust standard recommended amounts and those on certain medications for heart disease, depression, and ulcers may also have to adjust these amounts.

How to obtain the required amount of fluids

You can obtain fluids through other liquids besides water though not all liquids are created equal.

Stay away from caffeinated drinks like sodas, coffee, and tea. Caffeine is a diuretic and can cause you to become dehydrated.

It is also possible to get some of your water intake from fruits, vegetables, and the foods you eat. If you are eating an adequate amount of fruits and vegetables daily, then you are getting about one third of your daily water intake already.

High Blood Pressure: When the body is dehydrated, it limits the flow of blood to non-vital parts of the body in order to supply the vital organs with water. The immediate result is an increase in blood pressure.

Arthritis and joint pain: Cartilage is the slick cushion between our joints that allows them to move smoothly. Cartilage is made up of about 80% water. A lack of water negatively affects cartilage and increases the amount of friction on joints, causing early degeneration and arthritis. Discs along the spine and between vertebrae will also degenerate more quickly from a lack of water.

Digestion problems: Water is of prime importance in the gastrointestinal tract. It is the root of every fluid that our body requires for digestion. Without enough water the entire digestive system goes into panic mode and may cause indigestion, constipation, hemorrhoids, heartburn, and ulcers.

If you go for an eight hour period of time without emptying your bladder you are probably dehydrated. Other signs of dehydration include dark urine (it should be clear), an inability to focus, fatigue, crankiness, moodiness, dizziness, and headaches.

Scheduling your water consumption

Measure out your required water intake every morning. For example, if you have to consume 70 ounces of water a day, measure it out and keep that amount beside you in a glass jug. Drink from that jug throughout the day.

Though you will be getting fluids from what you eat and drink, trying your best to drink all the water in your jug will help you ensure that you get the amount of fluids that your body requires in a day.

Good reasons to drink plenty of water

Weight loss: Dehydration actually causes your body to secrete the hormone aldosterone that triggers water retention. Drinking more water releases the water that is being stored and allows weight loss to occur. Dehydration also causes the metabolism to work inefficiently.

Improves memory: The brain requires a lot of water because it is the only organ that is constantly active. Water helps it to maintain its constant level of activity. When water is lacking then the brains ability to perform slows down.

Water revives cells: Without an adequate amount of water, cells begin to suffer and die. Water restores a cells health and energy.

Exercise

Daily exercise is a very important part of the Mediterranean diet. Not only can it help you lose weight, but it can also radically transform your health.

Physical activity was a normal part of everyday life in the rural Mediterranean during the 1950's. Most people made a living farming the land or they grew their own food to feed their family. From sun up to sun down they worked hard in the field giving their bodies a complete and often strenuous workout.

This contrasts the typical American that spends five days a week in an office with little to no exercise. Exercise is penciled in after work for an hour or so and is given the flexibility to be bumped if a more important activity unexpectedly arises.

Statistics say that less than 10% of western adults exercise regularly. The American Heart Association, The Centers for Disease Control and Prevention, the Mayo Clinic, The Department of

Health and Human Services, and The American College of Sports Medicine all recommend getting a minimum of 30 minutes of moderately intense exercise every day in order to stay healthy and lengthen your lifespan.

The Journal of Experimental Biology states that sedentary people have a lifespan that is five years shorter than physically active people.

A low to moderately intense workout can include swimming, riding your bike, or going for a brisk walk. More intense exercise can include long distance running or high-energy sports, dance, or circuit training.

Understanding the importance of daily exercise is as simple as understanding the "use it or lose it" principle. If you don't use your body, you'll lose it. Without exercise your heart and lungs become less efficient which makes them more susceptible to disease. Your muscles become weak, your joints get stiff, and your flexibility lessens.

The benefits of regular exercise

Exercise prevents cancer: Studies show that a sedentary lifestyle, as well as diet are responsible for approximately 1/3 of cancer related deaths.

Exercise can reduce the risk of colon, breast, prostate, and endometrial cancer.

Exercise prevents heart disease and heart attacks: Cardiovascular disease is the number one cause of death in the United States. Fortunately, exercise can prevent it.

Your heart is a muscle. When you exercise on a regular basis your heart gets stronger, thicker, and more efficient. As the heart grows stronger, it beats fewer times. This allows the heart to *rest* more often.

A normal resting heart rate for an adult is between 60 and 100 beats per minute. An active person's heart rate is normally about 60-70 beats per minute or less. A lower heart rate is indicative of an efficient heart and good cardiovascular health. For example, an athlete's resting heart rate is typically about 40 beats per minute.

An inactive person's resting heart rate is about 80 or more beats per minute. The inactive person's heart has to work harder because it is inefficient and unconditioned. It can also only feed itself with oxygen between beats. The more the heart has to work the less time it has to rest.

Exercise keeps your blood pressure at a good level: High blood pressure is the most common type of cardiovascular disease. It affects 70 million American adults.

With every heart beat, the heart pumps blood through the body. The blood exerts a force on the walls of the blood vessels. This force is called blood pressure.

Things like stress, a lack of exercise, a high salt diet, and thick blood can cause resistance to blood flow, make the heart work harder, and put more pressure on the blood vessel walls. Any additional strain on the heart overtime increases the risk of heart attack and stroke.

Regular exercise keeps blood pressure low because blood vessels get bigger and more elastic when they are required to carry more blood during exercise. Bigger more elastic blood vessels make it easier for the heart to pump blood. It also helps to prevent clotting.

Exercise also strengthens the heart and cardiovascular system. A stronger heart can pump more blood with less effort. If your heart can work less hard to pump blood, the force on your arteries decreases, lowering your blood pressure.

Exercise lowers bad cholesterol and increases good cholesterol: If arteries or veins get obstructed by a buildup of bad cholesterol or fat, it becomes difficult for the heart to pump blood through the body.

Moderate intensity workouts can reduce the levels of bad LDL cholesterol and fat in the blood and arteries. This prevents the buildup of plaque and enables blood to flow well.

More intense workouts can raise the level of good HDL cholesterol and decrease triglycerides. This also helps to prevent the buildup of plaque in the arteries and it allows blood to keep flowing smoothly.

Exercise increases the production of red blood cells: Oxygen is transported throughout the body by red blood cells. Exercise causes the body to make more red blood cells so it can transport more oxygen faster.

Exercise reduces stress: Regular exercise decreases cortisol levels. This helps you feel less stressed. During exercise more serotonin (a positive mood regulator) is released. This calms you down.

Exercise also makes you happy. When you exercise, the body releases endorphins which are the body's natural opiates.

Exercise reduces depression: Exercise increases serotonin and dopamine levels which help relieve anxiety and depression.

Exercise improves immune function: People that regularly exercise get sick about half as often as people who do not exercise.

Exercise helps you lose weight: Your body keeps burning calories up to 24 hours after you stop exercising. Even when you stop moving, your body continues to burn calories.

If you exercise regularly your body will begin to use the same amount of energy at rest that others use when they're moving.

The extra oxygen that is created from exercise causes your cells to go into oxidation mode.

Oxidation is another word for burn. Instead of storing fat, your body begins burning fat due to the surplus of oxygen in your system.

Regular exercise also:

Prevents every major disease including diabetes

Helps to control blood sugar levels in diabetics

Prevents Alzheimer's and Parkinson's disease

Helps cleanse the body of waste and toxins
through perspiration

Improves the quality of sleep by turning serotonin
into melatonin which is tied to sleep patterns

Improves digestion

Strengthens muscles and bones

Keeps joints flexible

Maintains healthy bone density

Improves stamina

Increases tone, flexibility, and strength

Increases energy

Makes muscles thicker through the effect of
hypertrophy

Intercostal muscles and diaphragm get stronger

Cells become more sensitive to insulin so it can work more effectively

Promotes better balance

Prevents osteoporosis

The Mediterranean Diet Food Pyramid Daily, Weekly, Monthly

The Mediterranean diet food pyramid helps you make wise choices plus it's simple to follow. The bulk of the foods on the Mediterranean diet come from plants. Whole grains, vegetables, fruits, beans, legumes, nuts, seeds, herbs, spices, and olive oil are all daily requirements on the diet.

At the base of the pyramid are common staple foods that are to be consumed in large amounts and more frequently. Portion sizes and frequency decline as you go up the pyramid.

The pyramid is ordered in tiers that can help you plan your next meal. Each tier is categorized into either a daily, weekly, or monthly group that provides an idea of how often certain foods should be eaten. Tier one is the lowest and widest tier on the pyramid and tier nine is the highest and smallest tier.

Red wine is at the side of the Mediterranean diet pyramid indicating that red wine should be consumed daily in moderation.

DAILY

Tier One

Whole grains

At the very base of the pyramid are whole grains.

All whole grains start out as complete grain seeds of a plant. Each grain seed has three edible parts to it.

Bran: The bran is the outer, multi-layered skin of the seed. It contains fiber, antioxidants, B vitamins, and minerals.

Germ or seed: The germ is the embryo at the center of the endosperm. It has the ability to create a sprout. The germ contains unsaturated fats, protein, antioxidants, minerals, vitamin E, and many B vitamins.

Endosperm: The endosperm is the flesh that surrounds the germ. It provides the germ with the food and energy that it needs to sprout. It contains protein, complex carbohydrates, vitamins, and minerals.

Whole grains contain all three parts of the seed - the bran, the germ and the endosperm.

Years ago people would pick grains then grind them between stones to make flour. Nothing was taken away from or added to the grain.

In the late 1800's during the industrialization craze in America, a new method of milling and refining enabled manufacturers to remove the bran and germ from grain seeds. This created finer, whiter flour that was made up of the endosperm only.

The removal of the bran and germ got rid of fats in the outer layer of the seed that could go rancid. This enabled products to sit on grocery store shelves longer.

Refined grains like white flour, white bread, and white rice have lost about 25% of the protein naturally found in grain seeds. An additional 80% of other key nutrients have been lost in the refining process. Among these are essential B vitamins and fiber.

Over the years, processors started adding back some vitamins and minerals that were lost in the refining process. Most refined grains are typically *enriched* which means that nutrients like B vitamins and iron have been put back. Fiber however was not replaced.

Traditional Mediterranean food typically includes whole grains – the entire grain (the bran, germ and endosperm). Unfortunately, many Americans consume white breads, pasta's, rice, and other processed grains like doughnuts and rice cakes regularly that virtually have no nutritional value.

Whole grains are to be consumed daily on the Mediterranean diet. It is important to eat a variety of grains because different grains contain different sets of nutrients.

Whole grains such as amaranth, barley, bulgur, polenta (coarse cornmeal), buckwheat, brown rice, farro, kamut, millet, quinoa, wheat berries, whole grain breads, wild rice, whole grain pasta, and oats should be consumed at every meal in moderate amounts.

In the traditional Mediterranean diet, bread was a key part of every meal. A typical meal in some Mediterranean countries would include pasta, polenta, potatoes or rice along with fresh vegetables and legumes. In other Mediterranean countries it was common to have bulgur and rice served with vegetables, chickpeas, and various beans.

The health benefits of whole grains

Whole grains contain:

Iron which carries oxygen in the blood.

B vitamins that are essential for several biological functions.

Magnesium that is necessary for hundreds of processes in the body.

Selenium that helps regulate the thyroid and keeps the immune system strong.

Folic acid that assists the body in forming new cells.

Dietary fiber that improves cholesterol, helps prevent heart disease, stroke, type 2 diabetes, obesity, colon cancer, and rectal cancer. Fiber is associated with disease prevention because it enables the body to move substances through the body faster, giving the body little time to absorb them

Whole grains also contain other nutrients like flavonoids, lectins, beta-carotene, vitamin C, folate, phenolics, tocopherols, glutamine, oligosaccharides, and saponins that may lower cholesterol, help maintain a good blood sugar level, assist and improve the immune system, and help prevent disease.

How to choose whole grains

Read food labels: Look for a 100% whole grain or 100% whole wheat label on whole grain foods.

Look at the first ingredient: Choose whole grain foods that list one of the following ingredients first: whole wheat, whole grain barley, whole wheat bulgur, whole wheat rye, whole grain corn, whole oats, wild rice, brown rice

Look for the heart check mark: Since 1995 the American Heart Association has been making it easier for on-the-go consumers to make healthy food choices quickly.

Look for a white check mark in a red box on a whole grain food item. This check mark means:

More than half the grains in the product are whole grains

The product contains low trans fat, low saturated fat, low sugars, and low salt

The product does not contain hydrogenated oils

If you want to stay most true to Mediterranean tradition it is best to buy wholegrain flour and make your own bread and pasta. That way you can determine how much salt and sugar is added and you can rest assured that you are consuming the whole grain, the bran, germ and endosperm in order to receive the most nutrients from the grain.

8 servings of whole grains, brown rice, pasta, and breads are suggested daily

Tier Two

Vegetables, fruits, beans, legumes, nuts, seeds, herbs and spices

The traditional Mediterranean diet is a near-vegetarian diet. Its many health benefits are a direct result of the high proportion of vegetables and fruits that are consumed on the diet.

Several studies have examined the correlation between high vegetable and fruit consumption and chronic disease prevention.

Researchers John Potter, M.D., Ph.D and Kristi Steinmetz, Ph.D., R.D examined the relationship between vegetable and fruit consumption and the risk of cancer on 206 people and 22 animals. Through their research they found that cancer could potentially be a disease that is caused by low plant food consumption. They also found that eating vegetables and fruits raw seemed to offer the greatest protection from the disease.

The human body is better able to maintain good health and heal itself with a high consumption of plant foods. Studies have also found that consuming a high number of plant foods can help prevent, slow, or even reverse many other diseases such as Alzheimer's, heart disease, dementia, arthritis, and macular degeneration.

Vegetables and fruits have always been consumed daily by people living in Mediterranean regions. Vegetables are normally cooked or eaten raw drizzled with olive oil.

In the traditional Mediterranean diet, plant foods accompanied every meal. Fresh vegetables, fruits, salads, nuts, seeds and olives were consumed regularly along with fresh herbs, garlic, and onions.

Seasonal use of local or home grown vegetables would provide an abundance of antioxidants, dietary fiber, and micronutrients naturally found in plant foods.

Traditionally, many people in Mediterranean regions farmed their own land. Others had a manageable vegetable garden and fruit trees in their yard. Even people that lived in cities typically had window boxes in which they would grow their own foods.

For Mediterranean people, eating foods in season when nature intended, creates anticipation and allows them to live mindfully, and enjoy the moment. The richness of this experience has been obscured by American mega-marts that try to offer people whatever they want, whenever they want.

In order to stay true to the Mediterranean tradition it is best to shop for local produce or grow your own vegetables and fruits. Produce that is eaten in season shortly after harvest provides the most nutrients.

Traditional Mediterranean diet vegetables include: carrots, cabbage, eggplant, fennel, artichokes, mushrooms, pumpkin, sweet potatoes, shallots, radishes, leeks, kale, lettuce, okra, peas, beets, broccoli, Brussels sprouts, peppers, scallions, tomatoes, rutabaga, arugula, celery, collard greens, dandelion greens, cucumbers, mache, chicory, potatoes, spinach, turnips, zucchini, purslane, nettles, lemons, celeriac.

A variety of fresh plant foods should make up the bulk of your meals. Vegetables are full of fiber, phytochemicals, vitamins, minerals, selenium, and folate that help prevent disease.

Eating a few extra vegetables in a day is allowed because vegetables are high in nutrients and low in calories.

Each kind of vegetable has its own special collection of nutrients and phytochemicals, so it's important to eat a variety in order to get the most nutrients. Vegetables also have the most highly concentrated amounts of phytochemicals, vitamins, and minerals.

Fruits in Mediterranean regions are normally eaten daily for dessert although having both fruits and vegetables as snacks throughout the day is encouraged. Fruits are full of phytochemicals, fiber and essential vitamins (particularly vitamin C) and minerals.

Fruits common to Mediterranean tradition include: bananas, grapefruit, oranges, apricots, apples, pears, strawberries, blueberries, gooseberries, peaches, avocados, cherries, figs, grapes, nectarines, olives, dates, plums, melons, tangerines, pomegranates, clementines.

Tip: Choose organic vegetables and fruits. Eat one dark green vegetable and one orange vegetable every day if possible. Don't eat vegetables or fruits with added sugar, salt or fat.

The primary vegetarian sources of protein on the Mediterranean diet are legumes. These include chickpeas, black beans, white beans, green beans, peas, lentils, butter beans, fava beans, cannellini beans, kidney beans, lima beans, dried beans, alfalfa, licorice, and peanuts.

Legumes are low in calories and often replace meat in Mediterranean countries. They are full of vitamins, minerals, protein, fiber, and phytochemicals.

Nuts and seeds are normally used to add crunch and a punch of flavor to main meals, appetizers, raw foods, cooked foods, and dessert. They are packed with protein, fiber, phytochemicals, monounsaturated fat, antioxidants, and omega-3 fatty acids.

Studies have found that regular consumption of nuts and seeds can lower the risk of life-threatening diseases like heart disease and cancer.

Nuts and seeds that are common in the traditional Mediterranean diet include hazelnuts, pine nuts, walnuts, almonds, cashews, pecans, chestnuts, sesame seeds, pumpkin seeds, pistachios, and sunflower seeds.

Tip: Avoid packaged nuts and seeds that contain hydrogenated oils. This includes peanut butter and spreads.

Herbs and spices are also traditionally used in Mediterranean cuisine to replace salt and increase flavor. They have an intriguing place in Mediterranean culture as both medicine and food. They are also plant foods and therefore contain valuable nutrients and phytochemicals.

Salt is allowed on the Mediterranean diet but in smaller quantities than you might be used to.

Common herbs and spices include garlic, basil, oregano, parsley, thyme, mint, cloves, cumin, sage, pepper, fennel, bay leaf, anise, savory, rosemary, tarragon, lavender, marjoram, chiles, za'atar, sumac, and pul biber.

Quick fact: Garlic was primarily responsible for maintaining good blood pressure levels in Mediterranean countries during the Seven Countries Study due to its ability to dilate the blood vessels.

6 servings of vegetables are suggested daily

3 servings of fruit are suggested daily

2 ½ cups of legumes daily

1 ounce of nuts and seeds daily

Replace salt with herbs and spices

Tier Three

Olive Oil

Ever since the Greek goddess Athena gave the olive tree to the Athenians, olive oil and olives have been an integral part of the diet of Greeks and Mediterranean people.

Olive oil is at the core of the Mediterranean diet and is responsible for much of the Mediterranean diets health benefits. It is primarily used as the main source of dietary fat for baking, salad dressings, and cooking. Thousands of studies have been conducted on the benefits of olive oil in preventing disease. Researchers have found the following.

Olive oil supports cardiovascular health. In a study conducted on 200 healthy people in five European countries on the heart health benefits of polyphenols in olive oil, Dr. Maria-Isabel Covas, head of the Cardiovascular Risk and Nutrition Research Group in Spain found that those that consumed 25 mg/day of polyphenol rich olive oil had an increase in good cholesterol (HDL) that was directly related to the polyphenol content in the olive oil. She also found that lipid oxidation decreased (a major cause of cardiovascular disease) and that this decrease was an indirect result of the polyphenol content in olive oil.

Dr. Covas also found in several extensive studies on the health benefits of olive oil that people who consumed olive oil regularly had a lower risk of developing high blood pressure, high triglyceride levels, and stroke. She also found that a daily intake of olive oil reduced inflammation, reduced damage to the inner lining of blood vessels, and prevented blood clots.

Olive oil can help prevent strokes. A study conducted in France on 7000+ people over 5 years concluded that participants that avidly used olive oil lowered their risk of stroke by 41%.

Olive oil is effective against breast cancer. Oleocanthal is a natural phenolic compound found in olive oil that reduces inflammation which minimizes the risk of breast cancer. It also helps protect those in remission from getting cancer again. Scientists in Spain discovered that olive oil promotes tumor cell death and can affect the transmission of signals in the cells of breast tumors.

Olive oil can slow the hearts aging process. Over time our arteries may not work as well as they used to. A study conducted in Spain found that a diet rich in olive oil can improve arterial function in the elderly.

Olive oil can prevent type 2 diabetes. Spanish researchers found that a diet rich in olive oil lowers the risk of type 2 diabetes by 50%.

Olive oil can prevent osteoporosis. A study conducted in Egypt found that olive oil supplementation had a positive effect on bone thickness.

Olive oil can prevent Alzheimer's disease. A study published in the journal *Chemical Neuroscience* explained how a team of researchers examined whether oleocanthal could reduce the levels of beta-amyloid (the main cause of Alzheimer's disease) in the brains of lab mice. The researchers concluded that the oleocanthal in extra virgin olive oil can potentially lower the risk of Alzheimer's disease and dementia.

Olive oil has also been found to prevent skin cancer, colon cancer cell growth, metabolic syndrome, oxidative stress in the liver, ulcerative colitis, and loss of bone mass. Research continues to reveal more benefits of olive oil every day.

Olives are actually a stone fruit. Plums and cherries are also stone fruits. They are high in good fats, particularly monounsaturated fats, and they are a rich, nutritious source of 25 phytonutrients and important micronutrients. They contain no cholesterol and are low in carbohydrates and sodium.

Olive oil contains numerous bioactive and antioxidant components like phytosterols, vitamin E, and polyphenols. Polyphenols are antioxidants that allow the lining of the blood vessels to rest. This lowers blood pressure. Research has shown that consuming three tablespoons of olive oil daily can cut the need for blood pressure pills in half.

Olive oil is also one of the few culinary oils that has a fat content that is made up of 75% oleic acid. Oleic acid is a monounsaturated, omega-9 fatty acid that has a number of health benefits.

Oleic acid:

Helps to decrease blood pressure

Protects cell membranes from free radicals

Lowers LDL cholesterol

Raises HDL cholesterol

Burns fat

Helps to alleviate Type 2 diabetes

The combination of olive oil along with leafy green salads and vegetables is what is believed to give the Mediterranean diet its health advantage. The unsaturated fat in the olive oil paired with the nitrogen compounds in the greens and vegetables produce a new group of compounds called nitro fatty acids. Nitro fatty acids cause reactions that result in the dilation of blood vessels that in turn lower blood pressure.

In buying olive oil it is important to choose good quality fresh olive oil in order to receive the best health benefits that olive oil has to offer. Look for a green oil in a dark bottle. It will be expensive but fine quality extra virgin olive oil is well worth the price. People in Italy often have their own olive grove and make their own fresh stone pressed olive oil every year.

Olives are normally eaten whole and are used in the Mediterranean region for cooking and flavoring. Greek-style black ripe olives contain natural antioxidants that help reduce inflammation, fight cancer, maintain bone mass and promote heart health.

***2-3 tablespoons of good quality olive oil
are suggested daily***

Tier Four

Cheese and Yogurt

Dairy products have always been an important part of the traditional Mediterranean diet. They are consumed in much smaller quantities than plant foods, but a little goes a long way.

In the traditional Mediterranean diet, refrigeration was often lacking and the climate was normally hot, so milk was preserved and eaten as yogurt or cheese. Some milk was reserved for coffee or custard, but milk was never consumed as much as it is in the US.

Cheese was used to add depth and flavor to Mediterranean meals. Grating a small amount of cheese on a pasta dish was very typical as was grating a hard cheese like Romano or Parmesan over cooked vegetables. Serving a soft cheese like mozzarella with marinated vegetables and tomatoes, or crumbling feta on a Greek salad was also common. Creamier cheeses would often be stuffed inside pasta or vegetables.

Mediterranean dairy is unique in that it is made from sheep, buffalo, camel, or goat's milk. This kind of milk contains low amounts of animal fat.

Note: Animal fat can clog arteries and damage cardiovascular health.

If you think of the beautiful cheeses of France, Italy, and Spain you can see why dairy products have become indicative of Mediterranean cuisine.

The quality and flavor of the cheese was a luxury that far outweighed the quantity. A small cube of cheese after dinner was satisfying. Just savoring the flavor was enough.

The key to getting the nutrients that cheese offers without the fat is eating small quantities of it. Cheese can be high in saturated fat as well as sodium, but it is a great source of calcium.

The people in Mediterranean countries got some calcium from dairy, but more from plant foods like kale, almonds, figs, seeds etc.

The Mediterranean diet suggests that low-fat or nonfat dairy products be consumed daily. High-fat cheeses can be eaten monthly.

Yogurt was another form of dairy that was consumed on a daily basis on the traditional Mediterranean diet.

Tzatziki is an example of a typical way that Greeks would use yogurt. Yogurt was most common in the Middle East and Greece though many other Mediterranean countries also consumed yogurt regularly. Yogurt was also typically used as part of a pasta sauce, or as sour cream.

Greek yogurt is different from regular yogurt in that it is extensively strained to remove the liquid lactose sugar and whey. This gives Greek yogurt its thick consistency. Greek yogurt also contains double the protein of regular yogurt and significantly less sugar.

Other dairy products common to the Mediterranean region are brie, ricotta, Parmigiano-Reggiano, chevre, asiago, manouri, haloumi, manchego, and pecorino.

2 servings of low-fat dairy are suggested daily

1-2 servings of high-fat cheese can be eaten monthly

WEEKLY

Tier Five

Fish and seafood

The most common type of meat eaten on the Mediterranean diet is fish and a variety of seafood. This is due in part to the vastness of the Mediterranean Sea which makes seafood easily available, affordable, and always fresh.

Mediterranean fish markets daily display the catch of the day in order to provide their customers with the freshest fish and seafood available.

To stay true to the Mediterranean tradition it is best to buy seafood from your local fishmonger rather than packaged seafood from a supermarket. That way you will be getting the freshest fish from its natural habitat.

Every country in the Mediterranean region extensively uses seafood. Some of the most common and well-loved Mediterranean seafood dishes include paella which includes scallops, shrimp, lobster, and mussels; fish soup that includes a variety of fish and vegetables; baked or poached fish, and risotto with squid, clams, or shrimp.

Oily fish that are packed with protein and omega-3 oils are an important part of the Mediterranean diet. These oils are consumed in dangerously low amounts in North America and Britain.

Omega's are polyunsaturated fatty acids. They are called omega-3 essential fatty acids because the body needs them but can't make them. The only way to get omega-3 fatty acids is to consume them.

Two crucial types of omega-3's are EPA and DHA. These omega-3's are mostly found in cold water fatty fish. ALA is another kind of omega-3 oil contained in plants. Studies have found that ALA is not as potent a form of omega-3 as EPA and DHA although the body can successfully convert it to EPA and DHA at a slower rate. ALA is found in walnuts, flaxseed, and canola oil.

Omega-3's are crucial to the normal functioning of our bodies. They keep blood from clotting, help the heart maintain a regular rhythm, and prevent artery walls from hardening.

Studies have shown that eating even one fatty fish meal like salmon a week cuts the risk of heart attack in half.

Omega-3 fatty acids also regulate cholesterol triglyceride levels, prevent and alleviate joint pain and stiffness, ease arthritis, fight depression, promote bone health, help the circulatory system, prevent Alzheimer's, dementia, and certain kinds of cancers.

Fish and seafood common to the Mediterranean that contain omega-3's are salmon, tuna, sardines, oysters, shrimp, crab, clams, mussels, sea bass, eel, flounder, lobster, abalone, tilapia, squid, octopus, cockles, and whelk.

2 - 6 servings of fish and seafood are suggested per week

2 of those servings should be fish

Make 1 or both of the 2 servings of fish a fatty fish like salmon

Tier Six

Poultry

Poultry is the second most common meat eaten on the Mediterranean diet. It is an excellent source of protein that does not contain the high amounts of saturated fat that some red meats contain.

All of the Mediterranean countries use poultry in casseroles, stews, soups, and salads. A few bite-sized pieces of skinless chicken are often found in amongst a plate of whole grain pasta or rice and a variety of cooked vegetables.

There are of course dishes like chicken souvlaki where poultry takes more of the center stage in the meal.

In rural areas of the Mediterranean it is typical for people to have their own chickens in order to ensure freshness and make sure that their meat is not laden with chemicals.

In keeping with true Mediterranean tradition, buy free range organic chicken and eat skinless portions.

2-4 servings of poultry are suggested per week

Tier Seven

Eggs

The Mediterranean diet recommends eating eggs at least a couple times a week to a maximum of four times a week. This includes eggs used in cooking.

An egg is a complete meal in itself. It contains many of the necessary nutrients that the body needs. One egg is packed with 6 grams of high quality, complete protein. The protein is considered *complete* because it contains all 9 essential amino acids. One egg also contains 14 important nutrients including iron, folate, lutein, selenium, cholate, and vitamins A, D, E and B12.

Egg whites are almost entirely fat and cholesterol free so feel free to indulge.

One egg yolk contains 260 mg of dietary cholesterol. The recommended daily allowance according to the American Heart Association is 300 mg.

Cholesterol consumed in moderation is not as much of a culprit for heart disease as saturated fat. The latest research suggests that saturated fat is what you should watch out for.

One large egg contains about 6 grams of fat, 30% of which is saturated fat. Minimizing your saturated fat intake is the reason for limiting eggs on the Mediterranean diet.

When purchasing eggs, always buy free range organic eggs. You might even want to consider having a few chickens of your own in order to ensure that you are getting good quality eggs. Keeping chickens is inexpensive and doesn't take up much space.

The Mediterranean diet traditionally includes chicken, quail, and duck eggs.

2-4 eggs a week are suggested

Tier Eight

Sweets

The Mediterranean diet allows sweets on a weekly basis. Its philosophy is eat cake, but not as often and not as much.

Fruit is the most common dessert in Mediterranean countries. Fresh grapes are popular as well as any fruit that's in season. Sweeter, more decadent desserts are typically reserved for special occasions only.

Cannoli is a favorite Italian sweet treat from Sicily that is made with ricotta cheese, chocolate chips, sugar, flour, egg yolk, cinnamon etc. It can be enjoyed as a dessert or as a snack with coffee.

Baklava is a sweet, rich Greek pastry made of phyllo dough, nuts, cinnamon, honey etc. It is another famous dessert from the Mediterranean region that is traditionally only eaten on special occasions.

Gelato is another sweet pleasure that is synonymous with Italy. It is an Italian ice cream that is silkier and smoother than American ice cream.

Some of the best ice-cream in the world comes from the Mediterranean region. It is made with good products and without additives. Eating it is all about savoring the flavor.

Tiramisu is also a decadent Italian dessert that is made from mascarpone cheese, espresso, sugar, egg yolks, chocolate etc.

In Greece, the base of many sweet treats is honey and yogurt with a sprinkling of nuts.

Dark chocolate that is at least 70% cacao, or dried fruit (with no added sugar) are both nice options for dessert or as a snack.

The key to managing sweets on the Mediterranean diet is to think small. For Mediterranean people it's about the deeper pleasure of eating and savoring the taste.

1-2 servings of sweets are suggested per week

MONTHLY

Tier Nine

Meat

Meat is the highest tier on the Mediterranean diet pyramid.

Many well-loved Mediterranean recipes contain meat, but for people living in Mediterranean countries eating a traditional Mediterranean diet meat is consumed in very modest amounts.

The research done on the dietary patterns of the people of Crete, Greece, Spain, and Italy in the 1950's was at a point when poverty was high and farming was a way of life. People had to rely on their livestock for labor so to consider using them as sustenance was not an option.

Some common meat dishes in Mediterranean countries include roast lamb, moussaka made with ground lamb, veal shanks, or paella with chorizo sausage.

Holidays, special occasions and celebrations would often have meat as the center of the meal. Aside from this, meat was used in smaller amounts, about once a week in the traditional Mediterranean diet.

Make sure to choose organic, grass-fed lean cuts of meat in order to avoid the hormones, antibiotics, and GMO feed that is prevalent in lesser quality meat.

Meat common to the area includes: lamb, pork, goat, and beef.

1-4 servings of meat are suggested per month

Wine

Drinking red wine in moderation is encouraged on the Mediterranean diet pyramid.

A glass of red wine with a meal is common in Mediterranean countries where eating together and enjoying food are a couple of life's simple pleasures.

Research studies suggest that consuming red wine in moderation can reduce the risk of heart disease.

The cardiovascular benefits of red wine are due to the antioxidants from flavonoids that exist in the skin of grapes. These flavonoids lower bad cholesterol and increase good cholesterol. They also stop blood clots from forming.

The polyphenol in red wine called resveratrol also helps to prevent blood from clotting. Resveratrol exists in both white and red wine but red wine contains higher amounts due to the skin of red grapes. Also, during the making of red wine the wine stays in contact with the grape skins longer than white.

A recent article in the Journal of Nutritional Biochemistry stated that a moderate amount of red wine consumed daily reduces the risk of stroke (caused by blot clots) by 50%. The article also cited a 29 year study that revealed a 34% lower mortality rate among people that drank red wine daily versus those that didn't.

The effects of red wine on health have been studied extensively for many years. In addition to the heart health benefits of red wine, researchers have found the following.

Harvard Medical School researchers reported that red wine has anti-aging properties.

A team of scientists at the University of Leicester, UK found that red wine can prevent colon cancer.

Cedars-Sinai Medical Center in Los Angeles released a report that red wine can help prevent breast cancer.

Researchers at Loyola University School of Medicine found that drinking red wine in moderate amounts can lower the risk of developing dementia by 23%.

Hundreds more studies like these exist to support the benefits of red wine consumption.

In the Mediterranean diet a moderate amount of wine, typically one or two 5 ounce glasses of red wine served daily with a meal is suggested for men. One 5 ounce glass of red wine served with a meal is suggested for women.

Note: There are certain health conditions that may prevent you from drinking red wine regularly. If you have health conditions that you are currently dealing with or you take aspirin daily, talk to your doctor about whether daily red wine consumption is an option for you.

1 or 2 – 5 ounce glasses of wine are suggested daily for men

1 – 5 ounce glass of wine is suggested daily for women

Low Stress Living

Low stress living underpins the entire Mediterranean diet food pyramid.

The people of Crete in the 1950's and 1960's not only ate well, but they also knew how to take it easy, slow down and enjoy life. This aspect of their lifestyle had a very positive impact on their health.

How to alleviate stress

So, you know you need to live a low stress life, but how do you do that? Quit your job, move to a quiet Greek island and live off the land?

For most of us living in a fast-paced, money driven society, that's probably not an option. So instead, you can do things a little closer to home that will still make a significant difference. Here are some ideas.

Meditate: Find time each day to relieve stress through meditation. Meditation allows you to empty your mind and reconnect with your higher self. It frees you from stress by allowing you to fully embrace the present moment. As you consciously breathe in and out through your meditation, you are transported to a place of inner peace and quiet. Your body relaxes and you feel calm.

Exercise: Exercise is another great way to relax. It's amazing how much a brisk 30 minute walk can do for you in terms of clearing your head and bringing you back to a place of peace.

Meet with friends: Enjoy some time with friends. Whether it's going out for coffee or hosting a dinner party, savor the time you have together.

Journal: Expressing your thoughts, concerns, regrets, fears, and worries in a journal allows you to release your stress on paper. It also allows you to find clarity. As things become clear, anxiety and tension are lifted.

Be mindful: Being mindful involves allowing yourself to live in the present moment rather than battling between the regrets of the past and the worries of the future. It's about simple things like savoring your food, enjoying a sunset, listening to birds chirp, or enjoying a peaceful walk. Being conscious of every moment rather than being too busy to notice things in the present moment relieves stress. Mindfulness is also about acceptance. The more you learn to accept things, the less stress you experience.

Get a pet: Cats and dogs are great at helping you calm down and find peace. Just petting a cat or dog can lower stress immediately. Research studies show that pets can help lower blood pressure, improve your mood, and relieve stress. They also help with social support, alleviating loneliness, and providing unconditional love.

Laugh: You've heard the saying 'Laughter is the best medicine"... well, it's true! Laughter lowers stress hormones, stimulates circulation which causes muscles to relax, lowers blood pressure, and improves your overall sense of well-being. So, watch a funny movie, get together with your funniest friend or family member, or be light-hearted and turn day to day experiences into something funny rather than something serious.

Chapter 6

What is a Serving?

The Mediterranean diet encourages portion control. Overeating on good food can make you gain weight just as much as overeating on bad food can.

The USDA, American Heart Association, and Canada's Food Guide all publish serving sizes for various food groups. In general, here is what you can classify as ONE serving.

<u>Grains</u>

1 slice (70 calories) bread

1/2 cup (125 ml) cooked pasta, rice or couscous

3/4 cup (175 ml) whole grain sugar-free cooked cereal (like hot oatmeal)

30 grams whole grain sugar-free cold cereal

1 bagel, pita or bun

Vegetables

1 medium vegetable

1 cup (250 ml) raw leafy vegetables

1/2 cup (125 ml) other vegetables
chopped or cooked

1/2 cup (125 ml) vegetable juice

Fruits

1 medium fruit

1/2 cup (125 ml) raw, chopped, cooked or
canned fruit

1/2 cup pure fruit juice

Dairy

3/4 cup yogurt

1 1/2 ounces (50 grams) cheese

1 cup (250 ml) milk

Fish, Poultry, Meat, Dry Beans and Nuts

2-3 ounces cooked fish, shellfish, poultry or lean meat

1/2 cup cooked dry beans

1/3 cup tofu

1/4 cup shelled nuts and seeds

2 tablespoons peanut butter

Oils and Fats

2-3 tablespoons (30-45 ml) unsaturated fat

Serving sizes made easy

Serving sizes are often smaller than you think. In order to measure serving sizes properly, use these visuals.

1 cup - baseball

3/4 cup – tennis ball

1/2 cup – computer mouse

1/4 cup – one large egg

3 ounces – palm of your hand or deck of cards

1 ounce (2 tablespoons) – ping pong ball

1 tablespoon – a poker chip

Chapter 7

Why to Increase Good Fats and Decrease Bad Fats

The Mediterranean diet recognizes the importance of good fat. It suggests replacing bad fat with good fat in order to reap the many health benefits associated with good fats.

Over the years there's been a lot of talk about the importance of limiting fat in order to prevent disease, manage cholesterol, and lose weight. Doctors and nutritionists advocated a low-fat diet, but somehow a clear distinction failed to be made between good and bad fats. As a result people started cutting both good and bad fats from their diet.

Four kinds of dietary fat

There are four main dietary fats in the food we eat:

Monounsaturated fats

Polyunsaturated fats

Saturated fats

Trans fats

All fat is comprised of building blocks called fatty acids. It is the chemical structure of the fat that determines whether it is monounsaturated, polyunsaturated, or saturated fat. Some fats are a necessary part of a healthy diet while other fats can negatively affect our health.

Good fats are an excellent source of energy. They also support cell growth, provide energy, protect organs, help the body absorb nutrients, control weight, keep the body warm, manage moods, produce necessary hormones, and support brain health.

Both good and bad fat contain 9 calories per gram. This means that it's possible to gain weight with either type of fat. The Department of Health recommends that our daily fat intake should not exceed 35% of the energy intake we get from food.

Though the Mediterranean diet incorporates good fat it is not used in excess. It allows you to take advantage of the health benefits of good fats without weight gain.

When it comes to fats it's really all about what kind of fat you choose to eat and the amount. The idea is to replace bad fats with good ones and to stay within the daily recommended allowances.

Good Fats

Monounsaturated fats

All fats contain both saturated and unsaturated fat. The key is to choose fats that have a chemical structure that contains a higher proportion of unsaturated fatty acids.

Fat molecules that contain one unsaturated carbon bond per molecule are monounsaturated fats. These fats tend to be liquid at room temperature. Olive oil contains monounsaturated fat. It will only turn solid when chilled.

Health benefits of monounsaturated fats

Help lower blood pressure.

Help maintain good cholesterol levels (HDL) and decrease bad cholesterol levels (LDL). This lowers the risk of stroke and heart disease.

Provide nutrients that help the development and maintenance of cells.

Improve blood vessel function and help protect against plaque buildup in arteries.

According to the American Diabetes Association monounsaturated fats help reduce belly fat. They also help with general weight loss.

Monounsaturated fats lower the risk of breast cancer.

Some research shows that monounsaturated fats may help control insulin levels and blood sugar

Some monounsaturated fats like olive oil and olives contain antioxidants called polyphenols that help relieve pain and stiffness in joints caused by arthritis. They also help relieve migraines and lessen their frequency.

Oils that contain monounsaturated fats also provide a healthy dose of vitamin E. Vitamin E is an essential part of a healthy diet.

Good sources of monounsaturated fats

Monounsaturated fats can be found in olive oil, canola oil, peanut oil, tea seed oil, safflower oil, olives, avocados, nuts (almonds, pecans, macadamia, cashews, Brazil nuts, pine nuts, hazelnuts, pistachios, peanuts) nut butters, seeds (pumpkin, sunflower and sesame seeds), tahini, and natural peanut butter that contains only peanuts and salt.

Polyunsaturated fats

Fat molecules that contain more than one unsaturated carbon bond per molecule (double bond) are polyunsaturated fats. These fats are liquid at room temperature and only become solid when chilled.

The two main kinds of polyunsaturated fats are omega-3 and omega-6 fatty acids. The body is incapable of making these essential fatty acids and can only obtain them through food.

Health benefits of polyunsaturated fats

Help prevent heart disease and stroke.

Help raise good cholesterol (HDL) and lower bad cholesterol (LDL).

Help build cell membranes, maintain good muscle movement, and prevent blood clots.

A study in the Journal of Clinical Nutrition proved that consuming 4 grams of fish oil a day can lower triglycerides by up to 35%

Several studies have proven that polyunsaturated fats can help lower blood pressure.

May help prevent life-threatening heart rhythms from developing.

May reduce the risk of developing type 2 diabetes.

Ease joint pain caused by arthritis.

Support brain health and possibly help prevent dementia.

Some studies suggest that polyunsaturated fats can help improve depression and attention deficit hyperactivity disorder (ADHD).

Support child development during pregnancy and breastfeeding.

Good sources of polyunsaturated fats

Polyunsaturated fats can be found in salmon, herring, oysters, sardines, trout, tuna, anchovies, mackerel, walnuts, flaxseed, kale, spinach, parsley, seaweed, Brussels sprouts, olive oil, canola oil, soybean oil, sunflower oil, and corn oil.

How good fats can go bad

Heat, light and oxygen can damage good fats. Oils that contain high amounts of polyunsaturated fats have to be refrigerated and kept in a dark container. Flaxseed oil is an example of this kind of oil.

Don't use nuts, seeds or oils when they start to smell or taste bad.

Cooking oils on high heat can also quickly turn good fats into bad fat.

Bad Fats

Saturated Fats

Saturated fats are fat molecules that have no double bonds between carbon molecules. Instead they contain an excess of hydrogen molecules. These fats are normally solid at room temperature.

The biggest problem with saturated fats is that they raise the level of bad cholesterol (LDL) in the blood. If too much bad cholesterol builds up in the blood vessels it causes them to narrow. The occurrence of blood clots then becomes more prevalent and the risk of heart disease or stroke increases.

Sources of saturated fats

Saturated fats can be found in red meat, beef, pork, poultry with skin, lamb, butter, lard, whole milk, cream, cheese, fried foods, baked goods, and processed foods.

Trans Fats

Small amounts of trans fats are naturally found in meat and dairy products. It is the fake trans fats however that are considered the worst for our health.

Artificial trans fats are normal fat molecules that have been intentionally manipulated during a manmade invention called hydrogenation. During hydrogenation, heated vegetable oil is combined with hydrogen gas. This creates partially hydrogenated vegetable oil which makes food last longer on grocery store shelves.

Trans fats raise bad cholesterol levels and lower good cholesterol levels. Prolonging the shelf life of a product is great for manufacturers but it promotes inflammation, heart disease, stroke, and diabetes for us.

Trans fats can be found in processed food, fast food, pastries, cookies, and margarine.

The maximum daily amount of trans fat that the USDA suggests is 2 grams. Consuming less than that or none at all is better.

Trans fats may be identified as *partially hydrogenated oils* on some food labels. In the U.S., companies are allowed to label foods that contain 0.5 grams of trans fat per serving as 0 grams of trans fat. In order to determine if a product is truly free of trans fats you need to check the ingredients for *partially hydrogenated oil*. If this is on the label then there is trans fat in the product.

Due to misleading, yet legal labeling, you might be consuming more trans fat than you think since even small amounts of trans fat over time can add up to a lot.

Chapter 8

How to Choose the Best Quality Olive Oil

The entire Mediterranean region is filled with olive trees so it's no surprise that olive oil is the primary fat on the Mediterranean diet.

Olive oil is the oil that is released from olives when they are pressed. It's that simple. Press the olives and you get oil.

In a perfect world, every bottle of olive oil on the market would be naturally made by crushing olives and extracting the juice. Unfortunately not all olive oil is of the highest quality. There are various grades of olive oil that signify the quality of the oil.

Lower grade olive oil is extracted using various chemicals and is often diluted with cheap oils like soybean or canola oil.

Refined olive oil is extracted with solvents, treated with heat and adulterated with cheap oils.

Why choose "extra virgin" olive oil?

Extra virgin olive oil is the highest grade of olive oil on the market. High quality extra virgin olive oil is pressed immediately after harvest so as to get the best quality oil. The most sought after olive oil is extracted from olives using a method called cold pressing.

Modern production methods grind the olives gently so that heat is not created by the friction of the grinding. The temperature is carefully monitored during this process so that the olive pulp does not exceed 27 degrees. If the olive pulp exceeds 27 degrees then the olives can lose their flavor and the title "cold pressed" will no longer apply to the oil. This makes the oil lose its value.

Extra virgin olive oil is the oil that comes from the first pressing of the olives. This oil is considered the finest, purest, most nutrient-rich, freshest, and fruitiest flavored oil. It is the least processed olive oil and contains only 1% acid.

After the olive oil has been pressed it can be tasted like wine. This is how experts assess the quality, purity and flavor of the oil. Pure unfiltered oil is the most valuable. If the residues are filtered out then the oil is considered to be of a lesser grade.

In order for an extra virgin olive oil to be truly considered "extra virgin" the oil must be high in phenolic antioxidants, meet certain laboratory tests for acidity and peroxide levels, and taste like olives without exhibiting any flavors that would be considered defects by a tasting panel.

There are a wide variety of grades and flavors when it comes to olive oil. This is due to the different kinds of olives that are used together, as well as the region in which the olives were grown.

Greek olive oil can taste different than Tuscan olive oil and both can taste different than African or Italian olive oil.

Though extra virgin olive oil is the oil of choice, there is a lot of fraud on the market with oils claiming to be extra virgin when they are not.

Is it extra virgin olive oil?

So how do you recognize good quality extra virgin olive oil? Here are some tips:

Does the bottle have a label on it from the NAOOA (North American Olive Oil Association)? This trade group investigates olive oils to see if they really are what the manufacturer claims they are.

Look for extra virgin olive oils that are cold pressed with information on the label about where the oil was made (preferably a family run farm or company).

Check if the bottle has a harvest date on it as well as an expiry date. The closer to the harvest date, the fresher the oil. If there is no harvest date then you may be buying an oil that is rancid.

If you have a specialty olive oil store in your area that has a knowledgeable staff and offers tastings, shop there. If you don't, you can consider purchasing your olive oil from online vendors like *Olive Oil Lovers* (oliveoillovers.com) or *Zingerman's* (zingermans.com) that perform strict quality control in the selection of olive oils they choose to sell.

Don't be fooled by labels that say "bottled in Italy" on them, or that have a picture of a Greek or Spanish flag, or that have scenes from the Mediterranean countryside displayed. If there is no specific production point (mill) indicated on the bottle then it's probably not an oil worth buying.

Do your own test. Pour some olive oil on a white plate. Check the consistency. Is it thicker than vegetable oil? Does it smell like olives? When you taste it does it have a smooth feel to it and slight burn in your throat when you swallow? The burn is from the polyphenols in the oil.

A few more things to know when buying extra virgin olive oil

Olives are fruits, so consider olive oil a freshly squeezed fruit juice. That means it's perishable and tastes best the fresher it is. Make sure to keep your oil in a cool dark place and try to use up the bottle in one month. Also, make sure to check the label for the expiration date.

A bitter, strong and definite taste is a sign of the healthy antioxidants, polyphenols, and anti-inflammatories that are contained in the olive oil.

Asking what kind of olive oil you like is the same as asking what kind of wine you like. It's a personal choice and can best be determined by what you are using the oil for. For example the kind of olive oil you choose to dip bread into may differ in flavor from the kind of oil you want to use for a salad or cooking.

Light, oxygen and heat can make your olive oil deteriorate quickly.

Buy olive oil that is bottled in dark green glass. This helps filter out UV light that can cause the oil to go bad.

If you think that you will use up the oil within one month then make sure it is sealed well and store it in a cool, dark place. Olive oil should be used within one year of when it was made.

Extra virgin olive oil has a low smoke point and is best used in recipes that are cooked on low heat. Polyphenols in olive oil are compromised when heated.

Good olive oils come in various colors like gold, green and pale yellow.

Great quality olive oil can be quite expensive but well worth it because of the nutrient value that it contains.

Chapter 9

How to Switch to a Mediterranean Diet

Making the switch to a Mediterranean diet doesn't have to be difficult. First, lay a solid foundation for your success by understanding and accepting these four facts.

You're changing a habit

Change can be uncomfortable at first but it's worth it. It takes 21 days to form a habit so stick with it. Eventually, the Mediterranean way of eating will become natural for you.

It will take some work

Eating healthy takes time and planning. Let's face it, it's a lot easier to pick up a bag of chips or some take out than it is to plan healthy snacks and meals. The good news is that once you experience how great you look and feel as a result of eating healthy it will motivate you to keep going.

Creativity is key

One of the best ways to keep yourself motivated to eat healthy is to keep things interesting and exciting. Don't allow yourself to get bored with the food you're eating and don't expect anyone else to keep things interesting for you. Keep trying new recipes, serve food on fun, colorful plates, or invite friends over to try your latest Mediterranean recipe. Do whatever it takes to keep stimulating your interest. It will be well worth it.

Have definiteness of purpose

Napoleon Hill said that definiteness of purpose is the starting point of all achievement. If you know your "why" and you are committed to achieving it then the journey will be a lot easier and a lot more enjoyable.

Making the switch

In order for you to make a smooth transition to Mediterranean style eating, you need to go through the foods that are currently in your home and get rid of anything that doesn't fit the parameters of the Mediterranean diet. Starting with a clean slate will help your long term success.

The great thing about the Mediterranean diet is that the foods you need are readily available so you shouldn't have a problem stocking your pantry, fridge, or spice rack.

A couple other things to keep in mind are that you'll probably find yourself visiting the grocery store or local fishmonger more often than you use to. This is in order to get fresh ingredients for your meals.

You may also want to consider shopping the Mediterranean way by walking to the store, seeing what's fresh and planning your meals around that.

Prepare your home

To begin, browse your kitchen and pantry shelves and get rid of anything that is not in line with the Mediterranean diet. Margarine, processed foods, white bread, sugary cereals, and any oils that are not monounsaturated have to go.

Next, check the fridge and make sure that you've got the basics like farm fresh eggs, Greek yogurt, low-fat cheese, fruits and vegetables.

After that, have a look at your spice rack to see if you have what you need.

Also, check that you have a nice bottle of red wine on hand to enjoy with your meals.

Next, make sure that you have a good quality bottle of extra virgin olive oil on the shelf. Check the expiry date and try to use it up in a month after you open it. Keep it in a cool dark place after it's been opened.

Be a smart shopper

To fill out your kitchen shelves, pantry, fridge, and spice rack you'll probably have to do a little shopping. Here are some key things that you want to keep in mind when shopping for what you need.

Buy local and certified organic produce as often as possible. Shop at local farmers markets when they're available.

Buy local and certified organic dairy and free range eggs.

Make your own meals from scratch so that you can control the ingredients.

When shopping for spices try to buy spices that do not contain added salt.

Read labels: Be a smart shopper and watch out for things like hydrogenated vegetable oil. You don't want to see the word hydrogenated anywhere on the product that you are thinking of buying.

Watch out for a high amount of saturated and/or trans fats on the product that you are thinking of buying.

Beware of high amounts of glucose/fructose in a product. If either of those words are first on the ingredient list, the product is full of sugar, don't buy it. Also, beware of products that contain added sugars or preservatives.

Note: Words on an ingredient list that end in "ose' mean sugar.

Make sure that whole grain products actually say 100% whole grain somewhere on the packaging.

Buy canned goods that say "Non BPA Lining" on them.

Beware of an ingredient list that reads more like a science experiment than actual food. You want to recognize all or at least mostly all of the ingredients. Think of it this way. What would the ingredient list for a grapefruit look like? The only thing on the list would be grapefruit right? A simple, easy to understand ingredient list means a more natural product.

A word about leftovers

Don't reheat leftovers in anything other than glass containers. Leftovers can be kept in the fridge for 3-4 days. If you don't think that you can finish leftovers in that time it's best to freeze them right away because the longer you leave them in the fridge, the more the risk of food poisoning increases. Bacteria can exist on food without changing the taste, smell, or look of the food, so be careful.

Let's get started

The following list of supplies provides some suggestions to get you going. The items may vary from person to person but you can use this list as a general guideline. Feel free to take what you like and leave what you don't like.

Spices and Herbs

Allspice

Anise

Basil

Bay Leaves

Black peppercorn

Cardamom

Cayenne Pepper

Chili peppers

Chives

Cilantro

Cinnamon

Cloves

Coriander and coriander seeds

Crushed Red Pepper

Cumin and cumin seeds

Curry powder

Dill and dill seeds

Fennel seeds

Fenugreek leaves and seeds

Garlic bulbs

Garlic powder

Ginger

Lavender

Marjoram

Mint Leaves

Mustard seeds, dry mustard

Nutmeg

Onion Powder

Oregano

Paprika, sweet or smoked

Parsley

Pimento

Pul biber

Rosemary

Saffron

Sage

Savory

Sea Salt

Sesame seeds

Star Anise

Sumac

Tamarind

Tarragon

Thyme

Turmeric

Za'atar

Nuts and Seeds

Almonds

Chia seeds

Cashews

Chestnuts

Hazelnuts

Hemp seeds

Pecans

Pine nuts

Pistachios

Pumpkin seeds

Sesame seeds

Sunflower seeds

Walnuts

Legumes

Black beans

Butter beans

Cannellini beans

Chickpeas

Fava beans

Kidney beans

Lentils

Lima beans

Navy beans

Peanuts

Pinto beans

Split peas

White beans

Whole grains

Amaranth

Barley

Black rice

Brown rice

Buckwheat

Bulgur

Cornmeal

Couscous

Farro

Kamut

Millet

Quinoa

Rolled oats

Steel cut oats

Whole grain pastas

Canned goods and condiments

Almond butter

Black olives

Canned anchovies

Canned artichoke hearts

Canned oysters

Canned salmon

Canned sardines

Canned tuna

Capers

Diced tomatoes

Dijon mustard

Green olives

Kalamata olives

Ketchup

Organic salsa

Peanut butter
(made only with peanuts and salt)

Pesto

Pure maple syrup

Raw honey

Roasted red peppers

Sundried tomatoes

Tahini

Tomato paste

Tomato sauce

Worcestershire sauce

Oils and vinegars

Apple cider vinegar

Balsamic vinegar

Canola oil

Coconut oil

Cooking wine

Extra virgin olive oil

Grape seed oil

Red wine vinegar

Sesame oil

Walnut oil

White wine vinegar

Flours

Almond meal

Amaranth flour

Brown rice flour

Oat flour

Quinoa flour

Spelt flour

Whole wheat flour

Chapter 10

How to Make the Mediterranean Diet Part of Your Daily Life

In order to make the Mediterranean diet part of your daily life you need to start by keeping the pyramid serving suggestions in a place where you can see them. Here is a quick reference for you.

DAILY

8 servings of whole grains, brown rice, pasta, and breads

6 servings of vegetables

3 servings of fruit

2 ½ cups of legumes

1 ounce of nuts and seeds

2 servings of low-fat dairy

2-3 tablespoons of good quality olive oil

1 or 2 – 5 ounce glasses of wine for men

1 – 5 ounce glass of wine for women

Replace salt with herbs and spices

Drink plenty of water

Exercise for at least 30 minutes

Live a low stress lifestyle

Savor your food

<u>WEEKLY</u>

2 - 6 servings of fish and seafood
2 of those servings should be fish
Make 1 or both of the 2 servings of fish a fatty fish
like salmon

2-4 servings of poultry

2-4 eggs

1-2 servings of sweets

<u>MONTHLY</u>

1-4 servings of meat

1-2 servings high-fat cheese (optional)

Practical ways to incorporate the Mediterranean diet food groups into your daily life

As a general rule, you want to feature seasonal vegetables, whole grains, and fruit at every meal.

Whole grains

Cook up a batch of whole grains – bulgur, brown rice, barley, quinoa, couscous - and use a little at a time as a side dish for lunch, dinner, with vegetables, or in a salad.

Start your day with oatmeal, whole grain toast, whole grain pancakes, or a whole grain breakfast bar.

Have a sandwich, gyro, or bruschetta for lunch. Not only do you get your grains but you also get some vegetables too.

Try green peppers or tomatoes stuffed with brown rice, or try macaroni and cheese with whole grain macaroni.

Cut a whole grain pita into eight triangles. Place it on a baking sheet then drizzle it with olive oil. Season with pepper and a bit of salt then bake it at 375 degrees for about 10 minutes and..... voilà!...

pita chips! Serve them with homemade hummus and vegetables for a great snack!

Add barley to vegetable soup or stews.

Make a whole grain pilaf from brown rice, barley, wild rice, broth, and spices. Throw in some dried fruit and/or nuts of your choice!

Try rolled oats or steel cut oats as breading for chicken or fish.

Have a side of whole grain bread dipped in olive oil with your salad.

Snack on popcorn. Remember, corn is a grain, so popcorn counts toward your daily whole grain intake. Make sure to air-pop it and don't saturate it with butter. Instead, season it with garlic powder, parmesan cheese, and some olive oil. Yum!

These are just a few suggestions. Be creative and find your own unique ways to incorporate grains into your day.

Vegetables

In Crete, people didn't have to consciously think about getting six servings of vegetables into their day. Vegetables were such a staple that meals and snacks were automatically built around them.

If you think of vegetables as a staple then you'll have no problem getting them in. Remember to eat seasonal and certified organic vegetables as much as possible. Here are a few quick tips for getting veggies into your day.

Turn vegetables into snacks in the middle of the day, or get in the habit of having a vegetable platter on the table during dinner. Drizzle some olive oil over the vegetables before diving in and put a small bowl of nuts, seeds, and olives beside the vegetable platter so you can munch on those along with the vegetables.

Have a salad with every meal. Keep the salad simple with a handful of leafy greens, chopped tomato, crumbled feta cheese, and a dressing made of olive oil and lemon juice. You can jazz up this simple salad by adding peppers, carrots, sun-dried tomatoes, figs, olives, garlic, avocado, celery, cucumber, or any other kind of vegetable that you like. Nuts, seeds, herbs and even a sliced egg would also be a great addition.

Add vegetables to your current recipes. Put them in casseroles, stews, chili, and soup.

Make pasta sauce with chopped bell peppers, mushrooms, spinach, leeks, shredded carrot, celery, or green onions.

Put some eggplant, red onion, red pepper, tomatoes, mushrooms, and zucchini on a baking sheet. Drizzle olive oil over them and season with salt and pepper. Roast in the oven at 350 degrees for about 45 minutes. This is a great side dish that can be used with any meal.

Try a meatless Monday night. Build your meal around vegetables, whole grains, and beans.

Try skewered vegetables as a side dish. Use grape tomatoes, red onions, peppers, squash, or yams. Drizzle the skewers with olive oil and season them with a little sea salt, oregano, and cayenne pepper. Roast them in the oven until the vegetables are tender. Serve with a lemon wedge.

Slice some tomatoes and put them on a plate. Crumble some feta cheese and fresh basil over top then drizzle with olive oil.

Try a veggie pizza for lunch. Top a whole grain pita with tomato sauce, mushrooms, yellow pepper, garlic, zucchini, onion, and mozzarella cheese. Bake and serve.

Try some endive boats as a snack! Chop one apple, place it in a bowl and drizzle some lemon juice on it. Peel the endive leaves off and place them on a plate cup side up. Place some goat cheese, roasted almonds and the apple into the endive leaf and you've got a healthy endive boat for a snack!

Salsas are a great way to get a variety of vegetables at once. They make a great side dish or you can serve them with pita chips as a snack.

Steam some broccoli and cauliflower then make a sunny side up egg and serve it along with the vegetables for a healthy breakfast.

Change up your morning oatmeal by adding some cinnamon, honey, and canned pumpkin to it.

Try a spinach, mushroom, and cheese omelet for breakfast, some vegetable soup for lunch, and some roasted carrots and a leafy green salad for dinner.

There are so many great ways to get vegetables into your day. The more you consciously try to get them into your day, the more you'll become an expert at eating a lot of them on a daily basis.

Tip: Think of the colors of the rainbow when it comes to eating vegetables. The more colors you eat, the more of an array of antioxidants and vitamins you'll get.

Fruits

In Mediterranean countries, fruits are the grand finale to a healthy, delicious meal.

Fruits can be incorporated into your day as a dessert, main course, breakfast or snack. Here are some ideas on how to get more fruits into your day.

Simply have a peach, grapefruit, pineapple, apple, orange or any kind of fruit you like for dessert. Nothing complicated. Just one fruit just the way it is.

Add raisins, chopped apricots, pomegranate, or chopped figs to brown rice, quinoa or couscous.

Be creative and add fruit to your salads or top fish or chicken with fruit chutneys or fruit salsas.

Have an apple or pear with peanut butter or add apple slices to your chicken sandwich.

Pack fruits, vegetables, nuts and seeds for lunch at work.

A great dessert that you can change up a lot of different ways is plain Greek yogurt, fruit, toasted nuts and a little honey. First, toast some walnuts and pecans together and set them aside. Scoop about one tablespoon of plain Greek yogurt into a sundae dish then add any kind of chopped fruit that you like to it – raspberries, blueberries, strawberries, blackberries, peaches, pineapple, kiwi, papaya, pomegranate etc. Top that with a few toasted pecans and walnuts. Drizzle some honey on top then go to the next layer of yogurt, fruit, nuts and honey. Keep going in layers until you get to the top. Feel free to switch out the nuts for homemade granola if you like.

If you're used to seeing a cookie jar on the counter, remove the cookie jar and replace it with a bowl of fresh fruit. If you like your fruits cold put the bowl of fresh fruit in the middle of the largest shelf in the fridge right next to the milk. That way you will see an assortment of brightly colored chilled fruits ready to snack on whenever you're hungry. Use the cookie jar space for a bowl of fresh shelled nuts and a nutcracker.

The key to a successful diet is availability. If fruits and vegetables are easily accessible you'll likely get into the habit of eating those as opposed to unhealthy snacks.

Fruits are also great for breakfast. Place some olive oil in a non-stick skillet over medium heat. Slice a banana into rounds then place the rounds on a pan. Cook the banana rounds until they're soft. Serve them with any kind of breakfast item that you like, eggs, toast, oatmeal, pancakes etc.

Add fruits to whole grain sugar free breakfast cereals or oatmeal.

Top your waffles or pancakes with a variety of fruit or have a bowl of fresh fruit as the finale to a healthy breakfast.

If you have an apple or pear tree in your yard buy a dehydrator and dry the fruit after you've gotten your fill of eating it fresh. This is a great way to get dried organic fruit that has no sugar added to it.

There are so many different ways to consume fruits daily. A little creativity will take you a long way.

Fish and seafood

When it comes to seafood there is so much variety that choosing to eat fish and seafood two to six times a week should be an easy task.

Locate new recipes and begin to transition some of your beef nights into a fish and seafood night.

Make one night of the week a new seafood dish night.

Be creative and use fish and seafood in your main meals, in a sandwich, as a snack, in spreads or crumbled on salads.

If you need your transition to be a little more gradual, try a surf and turf night and reduce the amount of beef or "turf" to a single serving or half a serving size so that more of the seafood portions or "surf" are available to eat. This is one way to begin reducing your red meat intake.

Use seafood in chowder, casseroles, soup, pasta, lasagna and stew.

Use fish in spreads, crumbled into salads or snack on smoked salmon.

Bake, poach, grill or steam fish or seafood and serve it drizzled with some olive oil and a lemon wedge.

Remember that seafood includes scallops, clams, mussels, herring, lobster, crab, shrimp, squid, oysters etc.

Fish ranges from salmon, cod, halibut, tuna, sole, snapper, trout etc.

It's easy to get used to eating the same fish and seafood dishes over and over again but keep an open mind and try something that you've never tried before.

The main focus of your meals should be whole grains and vegetables. Fish and seafood should be seen as your primary source of meat and the add-on or flavoring to your meals.

The more you can change your thinking away from red meat and on to seafood the more you'll get in the habit of using it regularly from week to week.

Poultry

In between your fish and seafood meals incorporate some poultry.

Skinless chicken or turkey are fabulous additions to salads, soups, casseroles, pastas and spreads.

Strips of chicken are great served along with raw vegetables.

Use your choice of poultry in sandwiches that you can take to work with you.

Top pizzas with poultry and vegetables.

Use poultry for breakfast in omelets, frittatas or scrambled eggs.

Herbs and spices

In order to transition from salt to spices and herbs, begin introducing new flavors in your weekly dinner menus. Choose recipes that incorporate interesting exotic spices and include herbs in your salads, side dishes, spreads, dips and pasta dishes.

New spices and herbs are always great to try with cooked vegetables, legumes or in a vegetable dip.

You can even top your eggs with fresh herbs for breakfast.

Nuts and seeds

Nuts and seeds are great to snack on. They are an excellent alternative to chips, pretzels, and cookies.

Buy a few different kinds of nuts and seeds and mix them together along with raisins. Put them in a sealed glass container on your kitchen counter so that they are visible and easily accessible. You'll be more likely to eat them if you can see them.

Nuts and seeds are a wonderful addition to green salads, fruit salads and desserts. They're also great with vegetables.

Make your own toasted nut mix by putting some walnuts, almonds, pecans, pumpkin seeds, sunflower seeds and flaxseeds in a bowl. Drizzle some tamari (soy sauce) on top along with your choice of spices - cinnamon, turmeric, cumin etc. Toss everything together then pour the mixture out onto a baking sheet. Bake for about 20 minutes.

Use nuts as toppings for fish or chicken.

Pack some nuts and seeds in with your lunch.

Finely chop almonds and walnuts and add them to soup.

Try almond butter, cashew butter or pumpkin seed butter. Serve each with whole grain bread, fruits or vegetables.

Legumes

In order to get more legumes into your diet try the following ideas.

Include black beans in your morning omelet.

Use hummus as a sandwich spread or a dip.

Make chili and add a variety of beans like kidney beans, chickpeas and soy beans to it.

Add beans to your leafy green salads.

Include white kidney beans with any kind of pasta sauce.

Add cooked lentils to salads, quesadillas and soup.

Toast chickpeas and add them to salads.

Try some black beans seasoned with garlic, cumin and olive oil as a side dish.

Add some beans to your soups and whole grain dishes.

Olive oil

When it comes to olive oil always remember to dress, not drown. Olive oil can be used in a number of different ways.

Cook your scrambled eggs or omelet in olive oil, not butter.

Sauté your food in olive oil.

Spread some olive oil on whole grain bread.

Use olive oil as a dip for bread.

Drizzle olive oil on salads and on raw vegetables.

Make homemade salad dressings with olive oil. Try olive oil and lemon (or lime) for a basic dressing. You can change this basic dressing up several ways to keep things interesting. For example, try adding a couple tablespoons of white wine vinegar to it along with a teaspoon of Dijon mustard and some freshly squeezed orange juice. Or add a couple tablespoons of red wine vinegar to the olive oil, lemon/lime base along with a teaspoon of Dijon mustard, a few drops of sesame oil and some sesame seeds. As long as you have the base for a dressing, you can add anything else that you want to it.

Combine fresh basil, garlic, pine nuts, and some sea salt in a food processor. Turn on the processor and slowly add olive oil to the mixture. Keep pulsing the mixture until it has a thick consistency. You can use this quick, easy pesto as a spread, a pasta and on top of fish or chicken.

Use two parts olive oil to one part balsamic vinegar along with garlic, herbs of your choice, and salt and pepper. You can use this dressing on garden and pasta salads as well as cooked vegetables. You can also use this dressing as a marinade for meats.

Drizzle olive oil on meats and vegetables before baking them.

Combine olive oil with your choice of herbs and spices and serve as a dip for warm bread.

These are just a few ways that you can use olive oil from day to day. There are countless other ways as well. Always keep in mind though that olive oil does contain calories so go easy with it. Remember, you just need 2-3 tablespoons a day of good quality olive oil in order to take advantage of the heart-healthy benefits that it offers.

Dairy

Here are some quick tips for getting a couple servings of low-fat dairy into your day.

Have one cup of low-fat milk in the morning with a whole grain cereal.

Include some shredded low-fat cheese in your omelet.

Have some Greek yogurt and fruit for breakfast. Mix in some toasted nuts and a bit of honey if you like.

Shred some low-fat cheese on a garden salad for lunch or include a slice of cheese in your sandwich.

Try cottage cheese with raw vegetables.

Make a smoothie with lots of fruit, a couple bananas, plain Greek yogurt and some purified water.

Shave mozzarella cheese onto a pasta dish at dinner or into some homemade tomato soup.

Have a small cube of cheese after dinner.

Make homemade salad dressing using plain nonfat yogurt.

Top a pita pizza with mozzarella cheese or feta.

Put a vegetable platter and a plate of cheese slices on your kitchen table to snack on.

Try cheese and grapes together for a light snack.

Chapter 11

Tips to Supercharge Your Weight Loss

According to data collected by the Center for Disease Control and Prevention National Health and Nutrition Examination Survey 2011-2012 68.6% of American adults over the age of 20 are overweight. Of those, 34.9% are considered obese.

The BMI (Body Mass Index) is the most common way to assess the status of your current weight. If you have a body mass index over 29, research suggests that you are obese and at risk of developing serious health issues. If your BMI is between 25-29 you are considered overweight. A BMI between 19-24.9 is in a healthy range. A BMI under 19 is considered underweight.

So, what is the status of your current weight? Let's check.

Figuring out your BMI is easy. It just involves a bit of math. Here's how to do it:

Check what your current weight is in pounds and multiply that by 704.5. Next figure out what your current height is in inches then square that. Divide the number you got from your weight calculation with the squared number of your height. The number you get is your BMI.

Here's an example. If your current weight is 140 pounds then 140 pounds multiplied by 704.5 = 98630. If your height is 5 feet 5 inches then that is 65 inches. 65 squared = 4225. 98630 divided by 4225 = **23.34**. This is your BMI.

Quick tip 1: Enter "What is 5 feet 5 inches in inches" in a Google search to get the answer.

Quick tip 2: Enter "How much is 65 squared" in a Google search to get the answer.

Research suggests that the lower you are on the BMI index in the healthy range, between 19-24.9, the lower your risk of disease.

Now that you know how much weight you need to lose here are some general weight loss tips that will help you reach your goal weight.

Eat slowly

It takes about 20 minutes for your brain and stomach to realize that you are feeling full, so it's possible to dive into a meal and eat, eat, eat, then after about 20 minutes suddenly realize that you're stuffed. People that eat quickly are at more of a risk of overeating simply because they can eat more food in a shorter amount of time.

A study was conducted in 2008 on 30 healthy women that were asked on two different occasions to eat a meal at different speeds and then rate their experience on a scale that measured their hunger, desire to eat, thirst, satiety, and how much they enjoyed the meal. The study found that when the women ate slowly they consumed a lot fewer calories and drank a lot more water compared to when they ate their meal quickly. They also rated their feeling of satiety after eating the meal quickly lower than when they ate slowly.

A University of Rhode Island study found that eating slowly over 30 minutes can help you save 70 calories as opposed to eating in 10 minutes or less. That would enable you to lose about two pounds per month.

If you tend to eat quickly, do your best to slow down. Chew your food slower and savor the flavor. Designate about 20-30 minutes for each meal. This will allow you to enjoy your meal rather than feeling like you have to rush through it. Be mindful when you eat and focus on the food not on the TV, a newspaper, or your to-do list.

If slowing down is a struggle then try eating with chopsticks, a baby spoon or with your non-dominant hand.

Eat more fiber

Several studies have proven that adding more fiber to your diet will help you lose weight.

The great thing about the Mediterranean diet is that its entire foundation is fiber – vegetables, fruits, and whole grains. It is recommended that women consume 25 grams of fiber a day and that men consume 30 grams of fiber a day. Most Americans barely get half that.

Fiber helps you feel full longer which helps with weight loss. Also, unlike bad carbohydrates that pass through your body quickly and cause blood sugar spikes, fiber (a good carbohydrate) doesn't get broken down in your body rather it is absorbed by the digestive system. The soluble fiber absorbs water and forms a gel-like substance in your gut (like when you add water to oatmeal). This slows down how much sugar gets absorbed into your bloodstream. The less sugar there is in your blood, the lower your blood sugar level which means lower insulin levels which in turn means that your body is less likely to store fat.

Use smaller plates

When you decrease the size of your plate you automatically decrease your portion size without sacrificing the satisfaction of seeing a full plate of food in front of you. So, choose a smaller dinner plate, a smaller bowl, and smaller silverware. It's important to not feel deprived as you're changing your eating habits so using a plate or bowl that matches your serving size more accurately will help keep you motivated. A recent review of over 70 studies discovered that you can decrease your daily calories by 16% by doing this.

Split your plate into three sections

Visually split your plate in half then split one of those halves in two. This makes three sections....two small ones and one big one.

The big section is for vegetables and the two smaller sections are for your whole grains and protein.

You can use this as a measuring guide when you go out to eat or want to transition your dinner plate into healthier portions.

Practice smart snacking

See vegetables and fruits as snacks. Slice your vegetables into ready to eat snack sizes and wash your fruits when you bring them home from the store so that they are ready to grab as a quick snack when you're feeling hungry.

Keep a jar of mixed nuts on your kitchen counter and eat a handful of those along with your vegetable or fruit snack.

Prepackage snacks into portion sizes rather than eating from the full container. This can prevent overeating. When you pre-allocate how much of a snack you're going to eat then you're helping yourself stay disciplined.

Drink water before your meal

If you think you might have trouble sticking to your designated portion size per meal try drinking a full eight-ounce glass of water before you sit down to eat. Sometimes thirst can be mistaken for a feeling of hunger. Drinking a glass of water before you eat can get the digestion process started quicker which can help you stick to your allocated portion size during a meal.

Keep a food journal

Studies have found that writing down everything that you eat in a day can help you lose weight. In fact, one study showed that people who kept a food diary were able to lose twice as much weight as those who didn't track their food.

There is something significant about writing down and tracking our daily progress that helps us achieve our goals.

Prepare more meals at home

When you prepare you own meals you can control every ingredient that goes into the food that you're eating. This allows you to eat healthier, low-calorie, low-fat meals.

Also, when you're out and about, you're more likely to grab whatever's quick and convenient to curb your hunger. This means added calories and fats.

Relieve stress

Stress can make you gain weight. Your neuro-endocrine system gets into flight or flee mode when you're stressed and it deals with this stress by activating a hormonal signal to replenish your nutritional stores. This causes hunger. Since you're in a vulnerable state, your food choices may not be top notch. Also, the stress signals that your body releases can cause a buildup of visceral fat around your abdomen. This kind of fat is a silent killer and can lead to diabetes and heart disease.

Exercise

Do your best to get 30 minutes of exercise in every day. Remember that every minute of physical activity in your day counts and exercise in bits and pieces throughout your day is just as effective as exercise in one session.

Here are some tips on how to get more exercise into your day:

Take the stairs, not the elevator.

Park your car in the furthest parking spot from the store and walk. In fact, walk whenever and wherever you can. If you need a carton of milk and the grocery store is only three blocks away, don't drive there. Use this as an opportunity to get some exercise.

Lift and carry your own groceries.

Garden or do some heavy yard work.

Do family outings that involve physical activity.

Play with your kids in the park, go for a bike ride, or hike together.

Try tobogganing, cross country skiing or going for a walk on the beach.

Buy a pedometer and track how many steps you take in a day. Aim for 10,000 steps.

If you work from home and spend a lot of time on the computer, take mini-breaks throughout your day and try running quickly in place for one minute then go sit down. Get up again in half an hour and do thirty jumping jacks then sit down....or do twenty sit ups, or thirty step ups, or ten pushups. You can even just put some music on and dance. As long as you're moving you're exercising.

Remember, exercising does not always have to mean getting into your work out gear and going to the gym. We've made it too complicated. Keep it simple. Every bit of activity counts.

Get enough sleep

A lack of sleep can make you gain weight. Studies have shown that not getting enough sleep can slow the metabolism and make you burn calories slower. A Harvard study showed that even lacking a couple hours of sleep can cause the prefrontal cortex in the brain to be compromised. Since this part of the brain is responsible for self-control you could find yourself more susceptible to eating things you shouldn't be eating the next day.

Chapter 12

Mediterranean Myths and Facts

M. I'm a vegetarian so I can't eat a Mediterranean diet because it includes fish, poultry and red meat.

F. Actually, yes, you can still benefit from the Mediterranean diet. In fact, a lot of people living in Mediterranean countries in the 1950's and 1960's were vegetarian simply because they had to be. The main focus of the traditional Mediterranean diet is on plant foods. Yes, fish, poultry and meat are on the pyramid but that can be modified.

Whether you are vegetarian or vegan it is highly recommended that you meet with a registered dietician first to come up with a unique plan that will meet your nutritional and caloric needs. Because you will be excluding an entire food group and possibly some other Mediterranean diet foods like eggs and dairy then you'll want to make sure to get what you're missing from other foods.

M. The Mediterranean diet pyramid suggests that a lot of food be consumed in one day. Will I gain weight?

F. If you follow all the requirements of the Mediterranean diet you won't gain weight. That includes adequate water intake, daily exercise, and eating the required serving sizes per food group.

It can look like a lot of food at first but don't forget that serving sizes are surprisingly small. The Mediterranean diet is balanced so you get a little bit of a wide variety of foods every day.

The two biggest food groups on the Mediterranean diet pyramid (tier 1 and 2) contain the most amount of fiber. Eating a good amount of fiber every day helps you lose weight.

The Mediterranean diet is also low in fat (bad fats) and cuts out processed foods that are both sources of weight gain.

The fact that you will be eating a balanced diet full of healthy and nutritious foods, exercising daily, reducing your stress and enjoying life will all work together to promote weight loss.

M. *Coffee and tea are not allowed on the diet.*

F. Actually, coffee and tea are allowed on the diet. In fact, Mediterranean countries like Turkey are known for their Turkish coffee and Italy is known for its Italian espresso. Both tea and coffee are popular in Mediterranean countries. Tea, particularly herbal tea contains many antioxidants that are beneficial for the body.

If you drink a lot of tea in the evening or throughout the day you might want to consider limiting or entirely eliminating sugar. Drinking tea, especially caffeine-free tea, is like drinking water. It's like a mini-cleanse, so why ruin it with sugar? Sugar contains empty calories that you don't need when you're eating healthy and working to achieve your goal weight.

M. *I can eat fat-free and low-fat foods on the diet to help me lose weight faster.*

F. No. The Mediterranean diet encourages eating things like low-fat cheese and lean meats. It does not however encourage eating fad-type, fat-free or low-fat products. Many prepackaged fat-free or low-fat foods contain a lot of sugar, fillers, gums and other fake ingredients. Don't get sucked into marketing hype. Manufacturers know that words like fat-free and low-fat will influence your buying decisions. That is, if you're not smart enough to turn the package around and read the ingredients.

The Mediterranean diet focuses on whole, fresh foods and eating as close to nature as possible.

M. *The Mediterranean diet doesn't include game meat.*

F. Yes it does. Game meat was consumed in the traditional Mediterranean diet. It is not included in the pyramid because it is a less common food and normally harder to find.

If you enjoy game meat then fit it into the red meat category of the pyramid. Buffalo, deer, and elk are all lean meats.

M. *Those in the Mediterranean region eat huge meals and never gain weight.*

F. This is not true. If you want to lose weight then strictly following the Mediterranean diet can help you reach your goal. Mediterranean people are just as susceptible to gaining weight if they don't watch their portion sizes, don't eat right and don't exercise.

Chapter 13
7-Day Mediterranean Meal Plan

Monday

Breakfast

Mediterranean Breakfast Wrap.....1
(See Chapter 14 for recipe)

Plain Greek yogurt.....3/4 cup

Kiwi.....1

Snack

Fresh pear.....1

Low-fat cheese.....1 1/2 ounces

1 whole grain bun

Lunch

Whole grain bread.....1 slice

Salad made with:

....2 cups dark greens
(kale, spinach or arugula)

....strawberries - 4 ounces

....pecans – 1 ounce

....pumpkin seeds – 1 ounce

.....toasted chickpeas, 1/2 cup

.....black beans, 1/2 cup

.....fresh basil, 1/2 cup

.....salmon – 3 ounces
Season salmon with pepper and your choice of
spices. Cook in oven for 15-20 minutes.
Crumble the salmon over the salad.

Dressing:

....olive oil – 2 tablespoons

....juice of half a lemon

Snack

Cucumber.....1/2

Red pepper.....1/2

Unsalted peanuts.....1/2 cup

Dinner

Whole grain pasta.....2 ounces

Marinara sauce .....3/4 cup
Add onions, mushrooms, green peppers, olives,
tomato chunks, 2 garlic cloves, 1/4 cup cilantro

Whole grain bread.....1 slice

Drizzle with 1 teaspoon of olive oil

Red wine.....5 ounces

Dessert

Orange.....1 medium

Dark chocolate 70% cacao.....1 ounce

Tuesday

Breakfast

Whole grain bagel.....1 medium

Low-fat cheese.....1 1/2 ounces

Olive oil.....1 tablespoon

Pink grapefruit.....1/2

Snack

Whole almonds.....1 ounce

Sunflower seeds – 1 ounce

Carrots.....2

Lunch

Garbanzo Chicken Salad with Fresh Basil
1 serving *(See Chapter 14 for recipe)*

Whole grain bread.....1 slice

Dates.....1 ounce

Snack

Banana.....1

Whole grain bagel.....1

Peanut butter.....2 tablespoons

Low-fat milk.....1 cup

Dinner

Salmon, broiled.....3 ounces
Seasoned with fresh garlic, onion powder, black pepper and parsley

Brown rice.....1/2 cup, cooked

Brussels sprouts.....4 ounces
Can substitute with broccoli or asparagus

Zucchini.....2
Chop zucchini into fries, lay on a baking sheet, drizzle with olive oil, season with garlic salt and pepper

Peas.....1/2 cup

Whole grain bun.....1

Red wine.....5 ounces

Dessert

Apple.....1 medium

Wednesday

Breakfast

Bran muffin.....1 medium

Egg.....1 soft-boiled

Strawberry Greek yogurt.....3/4 cup

Peach.....1

Snack

Walnuts.....1 ounce

Red grapes.....1 cup

Lunch

Salmon Panzenella with Capers and Olives
1 serving *(See Chapter 14 for recipe)*

Whole grain bun.....1

Salad made with:

.....2 cups dark greens (kale, arugula, spinach)

.....red onion – 1 ounce

.....1 carrot – shredded

.....1 tomato – sliced

.....1/2 avocado - sliced

.....sesame seeds – 1/2 ounce

.....toasted chickpeas – 1/2 cup

..... Feta cheese – 1 ounce, crumbled

.....unsalted peanuts – 1/4 cup, crumbled

Dressing:

Olive oil and balsamic vinegar – 2 tablespoons

Snack

Black olives.....6

Pistachios.....1/2 ounce

Low-fat cheese.....1 1/2 ounces

Dinner

Brown rice - 8 ounces
Add 1/4 cup of chopped fresh tarragon and 1/4
cup pine nuts to the rice

.....peas – 1 cup

.....shrimp – 3 ounces
Add 2 fresh garlic cloves and 1 teaspoon of
fresh dill

.....olive oil – 3 tablespoons

Red wine.....5 ounces

Dessert

Fruit salad..... 3/4 cup

Thursday

Breakfast

Whole grain bread.....1

Almond butter.....2 tablespoons

Cinnamon.....sprinkle on bread

Banana.....1

Apple.....1

Snack

Hummus.....1/2 cup

Cucumber.....1/2

Celery.....2 sticks

Pita chips.....1 pita

Lunch

1 cup couscous
Add tomato, yellow pepper, onion, zucchini and
fresh parsley

Salmon - 3 ounces
Season with pepper, garlic powder and cumin
Cook in oven for 20 minutes

Steamed broccoli.....1/2 cup

Asparagus.....4 stems
Pour 1 tablespoon olive oil on pan, add asparagus.
Cook until soft.

Snack

Pecans.....1 ounce

Unsalted peanuts.....1 ounce

Green grapes.....4 ounces

Dinner

Mediterranean Creamy Panini.....1 serving
(See Chapter 14 for recipe)

Red wine.....5 ounces

Dessert

Orange.....1 medium

Vanilla Greek yogurt.....2 ounces

Friday

Breakfast

Unrefined whole grain cereal.....1 cup

Almond milk....1 cup

Raspberries.....1/4 cup, sliced

Snack

Fresh pineapple.....3 sliced rings

Macadamia nuts.....1 ounce

Sunflower seeds.....1/2 ounce

Lunch

Whole wheat pita.....1 ounce filled with:
1/2 cup anchovies, chopped onion, black olives,
celery, 1/8 cup black beans and 2 tablespoons
Greek Tzatziki sauce

Carrot.....1 stick

Snack

Whole grain bread....1 slice

Avocado.....1/2

Tomato.....1/2

Dinner

Roasted Bell Pepper and Artichoke Pasta
Salad.....1 serving
(See Chapter 14 for recipe)

Mushrooms.....1/2 cup
Sautéed in olive oil, with fresh garlic, fresh basil,
green onions, 1/2 cup peas

Barley bread.....2 ounces

Red wine.....5 ounces

Dessert

Cherries.....1/4 cup

Saturday

Breakfast

Blueberry muffin.....1

Egg.....1 soft-boiled

Strawberries.....1/4 cup, sliced

Low-fat milk.....1 cup

Snack

Yellow pepper.....1/2

Celery sticks.....2

Radish.....1 ounce

Hummus.....1/2 cup

Lunch

Greek Salad with Chicken – 1 serving
(*See Chapter 14 for recipe*)

Snack

Whole grain bread.....1 slice

Cashew butter.....2 tablespoons

Banana.....1

Dinner

Baked potato.....1
Topped with steamed zucchini, broccoli, mushrooms, cauliflower, asparagus, green beans, fresh dill, scallions, black pepper. Drizzle with olive oil.

Cod....3 ounces
Season with pepper and garlic powder. Dip in egg, flour and bread crumbs. Bake in oven for 15 minutes.

Whole grain bun.....1

Red wine.....5 ounces

Dessert

Fruit salad made with:

.....Banana.....1 medium

.....Kiwi.....1

.....Strawberries.....2 ounces

.....Blueberries.....2 ounces

.....Pomegranate.....1/2

Drizzle with 1 teaspoon of honey

Sunday

Breakfast

Whole grain English muffin.....1

Plain Greek yogurt.....3/4 cup topped with:

.....toasted pecans and walnuts 1 ounce

..... mixed berries

Snack

Dates.....1 ounce

Lunch

Whole grain bread.....2 ounces

Salad made with:

.....2 cups dark greens – kale or spinach

.....endive - 1 sliced

.....red onion - 1 slice

.....jicama – 1/2 cup, matchsticks

.....sunflower seeds – 2 tablespoons

.....goat cheese, crumbled

Dressing:

....olive oil −2 tablespoons

....juice of 1 lime

Snack

Broccoli.....1/4 cup

Cauliflower.....1/4 cup

Hummus.....1/2 cup

Dinner

Garlic Linguine.....1 serving
(*See Chapter 14 for recipe*)

Salad made with:

.....spinach - 2 cups

..... red onion − 2 slices

......orange − 1 sliced

.....alfalfa − 1/2 cup

.....pumpkin seeds.....1 ounce

Dressing:

.....olive oil - 2 tablespoons

.....red wine vinegar – 1 tablespoon

.....whole grain mustard – 1 teaspoon

.....orange juice – 2 tablespoons

.....chopped fresh cilantro – 1 /8 cup

.....sesame oil – 2 tablespoons

Red wine.....5 ounces

Dessert

Pink grapefruit.....1/2

Dark chocolate 70% cacao.....1 ounce

Chapter 14

30 Minute Mediterranean Diet Recipes

Find more delicious 30 minute recipes in my Mediterranean Diet Cookbook

Available on Amazon

Mediterranean Breakfast Wrap

Prep time: 15 minutes

Makes 2 wraps

Ingredients

Eggs.....4 large

Yellow onion.....1/4 cup

Sweet red pepper.....1/4 cup

Tomato.....1 small, chopped

Fresh baby spinach.....1/2 cup, torn

Fresh basil....1 teaspoon, chopped

Whole wheat tortillas.....2 (7-8 inches)

Low-fat feta-cheese.....1 ounce, crumbled

Extra virgin olive oil.....3 tablespoons

Salt.....1/8 teaspoon

Black pepper....1/4 teaspoon

Directions

Heat the olive oil in a non-stick pan. Add the onion and sweet red pepper to it and cook over medium heat until both are soft. Add the eggs and fresh basil. Season with salt and pepper then let the eggs set.

Place the baby spinach and tomato in the center of each whole wheat tortilla then add the egg mixture and top with feta cheese. Fold and serve.

Vegetable Omelet with Fennel

Serves 4

Ingredients

Eggs.....6

Fennel bulb.....2 cups, thinly sliced

Cherry tomatoes.....8 sliced

Green brine-cured olives.....1/4 cup, pitted and chopped

Artichoke hearts.....1/4 cup, marinated in water, rinsed, drained and chopped

Goat cheese.....1/2 cup, crumbled

Fresh dill, basil or parsley.....2 tablespoons, chopped

Extra virgin olive oil.....1 tablespoon

Salt.....1/4 teaspoon

Black pepper.....1/2 teaspoon

Directions

Preheat the oven to 350 degrees.

In a skillet, heat the olive oil over medium high heat and sauté the fennel for five minutes.

Add the artichokes, tomatoes and olives to the pan. Sauté for another three minutes or until the artichokes soften.

In a large bowl, whisk the eggs, salt and pepper together.

Pour the whisked egg mixture into the skillet over the vegetables and stir for a couple of minutes.

Sprinkle the crumbled goat cheese on top and place into oven. Bake for five minutes. Check to see if the eggs are cooked through by inserting a knife or fork through the center. It should come out clean of any liquid.

Remove from the oven and allow the dish to set for one minute. Cut into four wedges.

Top with dill, basil or parsley and serve.

Rise and Shine Chickpea, Zucchini Hash Browns

Serves 4

Ingredients

Sweet potatoes.....4 cups, shredded

Chickpeas.....1-15 ounce can, rinsed

Baby spinach.....2 cups, chopped

Zucchini.....1 cup, chopped

Yellow onion.....1/3 cup, chopped

Eggs.....4 large

Curry powder.....1 tablespoon

Fresh ginger.....1 tablespoon, minced

Extra virgin olive oil.....1/4 cup

Fresh garlic.....1 clove

Salt.....1/2 teaspoon

Black pepper.....1/2 teaspoon

Directions

In a large bowl, combine the sweet potatoes, baby spinach, onion, curry powder, ginger, salt and pepper.

Heat the oil in a large pan over medium heat. Add the potato mixture and press down so that the potatoes cover the pan in a single layer. Allow them to cook over medium heat for five minutes.

Lower the heat and add the chickpeas, zucchini and garlic. Break up the potatoes a bit to combine then press down again into a single layer.

Make four nests in the potato mixture. Crack one egg into each nest and cook for five minutes until the eggs have set. Serve.

Ratatouille

Ingredients

Eggplant.....1 peeled, cut into 1 inch cubes

Yellow onion.....1 medium, chopped

Zucchini.....1 cut into 1 inch cubes

Tomatoes.....1 – 15 ounce can

Fresh basil.....1/2 cup, chopped

Black olives.....1/2 cup, pitted and chopped

Yellow bell pepper.....1 large, diced

Red bell pepper.....1 large, diced

Fresh garlic.....4 cloves, finely chopped

Extra virgin olive oil.....7 tablespoons, divided

Cayenne pepper.....1/2 teaspoon

Sea salt.....2 teaspoons

Sugar.....1 teaspoon

Directions

Place a colander in the sink and put the one inch cubes of eggplant in it. Season the eggplant with sea salt and toss. Weigh the eggplant down with a bowl. This will allow the juices to drain into the sink.

Heat two tablespoons of oil in a nonstick pan over low to medium heat. Add the peppers, garlic and onion and sauté. Remove from the pan and place into a medium bowl.

Add three tablespoons of oil to the pan along with the eggplant cubes. Sauté the eggplant until it is soft. Remove from the pan and add the eggplant to the peppers mixture.

Add two tablespoons of oil to the pan and sauté the zucchini until it is soft. Remove from pan and add it to the peppers and eggplant mixture.

Add the tomatoes and sugar to the pan along with the cayenne pepper. Simmer and stir often until the tomatoes thicken. Add the peppers and eggplant mixture to the pan. Warm through then add the basil and olives. Serve with rice. Enjoy!

Shrimp in White Wine with Penne Pasta

Serves 8

Ingredients

Penne pasta.....1 - 16 ounce package

Red onion.....1/4 cup, chopped

Garlic.....1 tablespoon, chopped

White wine.....1/4 cup

Tomatoes.....3 - 14.5 ounce can, diced

Shrimp.....1 pound, peeled and deveined

Parmesan cheese.....1 cup, grated

Extra virgin olive oil.....2 tablespoons

Salt.....1 teaspoon

Directions

Fill a large pot three quarters full of water and add one teaspoon of salt to it. Bring it to a boil and add the penne pasta. Check the pasta within eight to ten minutes. The pasta will be done when it is al dente, slightly firm.

While the pasta is boiling, heat two tablespoons of olive oil in a medium saucepan over medium heat.

Add the red onion and garlic. Cook until the onions are opaque and the garlic is toasted.

Add the tomatoes and white wine and mix well. Reduce to simmer and let the flavors marinate for ten minutes stirring occasionally.

Add the shrimp to the skillet and let it cook for five to seven minutes.

Drain the pasta and return it to the large pot.

Take the cooked ingredients in the skillet and add it to the large pasta pot. Mix and serve hot with grated parmesan cheese.

Salmon Panzanella with Capers and Olives

Serves 4

Ingredients

Fresh salmon.....1 pound, skinned and cut into four sections

Kalamata olives.....8 pitted and chopped

Red wine vinegar.....3 tablespoons

Tomatoes.....2 cut into one inch pieces

Cucumber.....1 medium, seeded and peeled, cut into one inch slices

Whole grain bread.....3 thick slices, toasted, cut into one inch cubes

Capers.....1 tablespoon, rinsed and chopped

Red onion.....1 thinly sliced

Fresh basil.....1/2 cup, chopped

Extra virgin olive oil.....3 tablespoons

Black pepper.....1/2 teaspoon, divided

Salt..... 1/2 teaspoon

Directions

Preheat the oven to 300 degrees or prepare the grill.

In a bowl, whisk together the olives, red wine vinegar, capers and half the black pepper. Slowly whisk in the olive oil. Add the bread, cucumbers, tomatoes, onion and basil.

Oil the grill or baking dish to avoid sticking.

Season both sides of the salmon with the remaining black pepper and salt. Broil or grill the salmon for about five minutes on each side until the fish flakes.

Gently mix the ingredients in the bowl and place it on individual serving platters. Top with broiled or grilled fish fillets and serve immediately.

Roasted Bell Pepper and Artichoke Pasta Salad

Serves 4

Ingredients

Farfalle.....8 ounces, whole grain

Artichoke hearts.....1 can - 13.5 ounces in water, drained and chopped

Mozzarella cheese.....8 ounces, partly skimmed, shredded

Roasted bell peppers.....1/4 cup bottled, chopped

Peas.....1/2 cup, frozen

Fresh parsley.....1/4 cup, chopped

Juice and zest of 1 lemon

Extra virgin olive oil.....2 teaspoons

Directions

Cook the farfalle according to the package directions, omitting any salt or added fats.

While the pasta cooks, combine the lemon zest, lemon juice and olive oil in a large bowl then whisk.

Add artichoke hearts, bell pepper, cheese, and parsley to it. Toss to combine.

Place the peas in a colander. Drain the pasta over the peas in the colander. Shake well but do not run water over the pasta.

Add the pasta and peas to the large bowl with the lemon mixture. Toss to combine. Serve warm or at room temperature.

Greek Salad with Chicken

Serves 4

Ingredients

Chicken.....2 ½ cups, cooked and chilled (about 12 ounces)

Romaine lettuce.....6 cups, chopped

Tomatoes.....2 chopped

Cucumber.....1 medium, chopped

Black olives.....1/2 cup, pitted and sliced

Feta cheese.....1/2 cup

Red onion.....1/2 cup, finely chopped

Fresh dill or oregano.....1 tablespoon, chopped

Garlic powder.....1 teaspoon

Red wine vinegar.....1/3 cup

Extra virgin olive oil.....2 tablespoons

Salt.....1/4 teaspoon

Black pepper.....1/4 teaspoon

Directions

In a large bowl, whisk together the red-wine vinegar, olive oil, dill or oregano, garlic powder and salt and pepper.

Add chicken, lettuce, tomatoes, cucumber, red onion, olives, and feta cheese. Stir together and serve on chilled plates.

Mediterranean Style Portobello Mushrooms

Serves 6

Ingredients

Italian sausage.....4 ounces

Portobello mushrooms.....8

Celery.....1 stalk, chopped

Whole-grain bread.....4 slices

White onion.....1/2 cup, finely chopped

Garlic.....4 cloves, chopped

Ground sage.....3/4 teaspoon

Caraway seeds.....3/4 teaspoon

Parmesan.....6 tablespoons, grated

Extra virgin olive oil.....6 tablespoons, divided

Salt.....dash

Directions

Brush two tablespoons of olive oil onto a baking sheet. Place six of the eight portobellos onto the baking sheet and warm them in a 250 degree oven for about ten minutes.

Toast the whole-grain bread then chop it into small cubes. Set aside.

Chop the remaining two portobellos and set them aside.

Heat a nonstick pan with two tablespoons of olive oil. Add the Italian sausage and chopped portobellos. Heat through. Add the sage, caraway seeds and bread. Stir. Remove the mixture and place into a bowl.

Add the remaining two tablespoons of olive oil to the pan along with the garlic, celery and onion. Sauté until soft. Remove from pan and add to the sausage mixture. Toss together.

Set the oven to 400 degrees. Stuff each portobello with the sausage mixture. Top each with a dash of salt and one tablespoon of parmesan.

Cook portobellos for about 15 minutes until they have heated through and the cheese has slightly browned. Serve.

Garlic Linguine

Serves 4

Ingredients

Linguine.....8 ounces

Tomatoes.....2 cups, chopped

Garlic.....2 teaspoons, minced

Basil.....1 tablespoon, dried

Oregano.....1 tablespoon, dried

Thyme.....1 teaspoon, dried

Fresh Parsley.....2 tablespoons, chopped

Extra virgin olive oil.....2 tablespoons

Directions

Fill a large pasta pot three quarters full of water and boil.

Add pasta to the boiling water and cook until it reaches your desired level of tenderness.

Add olive oil to a large saucepan over medium heat.

Add the garlic, basil, oregano, and thyme to the saucepan and stir.

When the linguine is cooked, add it to the large saucepan with the garlic and herbs. Mix well. Add the tomatoes and stir until the ingredients are well combined.

Remove from heat. Top with fresh parsley and serve immediately.

Mediterranean Creamy Panini

Serves 4

Ingredients

Whole grain bread.....8 slices

Romaine lettuce.....8 leaves

Zucchini.....1 small, thinly sliced

Tomato.....1 sliced

Provolone cheese.....4 slices

Roasted red peppers.....1 jar, drained and sliced

Bacon.....8 slices, cooked

Fresh basil.....1/4 cup, chopped

Black olives.....2 tablespoons, pitted and chopped

Homemade Mayonnaise.....1/4 cup

Extra virgin olive oil.....1 tablespoon

Homemade mayonnaise

Makes 3/4 cups of mayo

Egg.....1 large, egg yolk only

1 ½ teaspoons fresh lemon juice

White wine vinegar.....1 teaspoon

Dijon mustard.....1/2 teaspoon

Extra virgin olive oil.....3/4 cup

Combine all the ingredients in a medium bowl. Whisk until blended. Add a 1/4 cup of the olive oil to the mixture a few drops at a time. Slowly add the remaining 1/2 cup of olive oil whisking constantly. Cover and put in refrigerator.

Directions

In a medium skillet on medium heat, cook the bacon until it's done. Remove the bacon and place it on some paper towel to reduce the fat drippings.

In a small bowl, combine the mayonnaise, black olives and basil.

Spread the mayonnaise mixture on each slice of bread. Add two slices of tomato, sliced zucchini, peppers, provolone, two bacon strips, and one lettuce leaf then cover with another piece of bread. Repeat three times to make the other sandwiches.

Heat 1 tablespoon of olive oil in a large skillet on medium heat. Place the sandwiches in the skillet to brown the bread, about five minutes each side.

Cut the sandwiches in half and serve immediately.

Pan Seared Salmon with Dill Sauce, Fennel and Red Wine

Serves 4

Ingredients

Tomato.....1 large, chopped

Fennel.....1 cup, finely chopped (about 1/2 bulk stalks, trimmed)

Red onion.....2 tablespoons, chopped

Dill....2 tablespoons, minced

Red wine vinegar.....1 tablespoon

Salt.....1/2 teaspoon, divided

Salmon fillet.....1 pound, skinned

Extra virgin olive oil.....2 tablespoons

Black pepper to taste

Directions

In a medium bowl, combine the tomato, fennel, red onion, dill, red-wine vinegar and a dash of salt. Set aside.

Cut the salmon fillets into four portions. Sprinkle the front and back of the fillets with the remaining salt and pepper.

In a medium skillet on high heat, add the olive oil. It should be shimmering but not smoking.

Add the salmon skin side up and brown, about three to five minutes. Turn the salmon over to brown the other side. Remove pan from heat and allow the salmon to continue to cook through, about three to five minutes.

Plate the salmon and top with the salsa. Serve immediately.

Roasted Cod with Olive-Caper Tapenade

Serves 4

Ingredients

Cod fillets.....1 ½ pounds

Cherry tomatoes.....1 ½ cups, halved

Kalamata olives.....1/2 cup, chopped

Capers.....2 tablespoons

Fresh oregano.....2 ½ teaspoons

Shallot.....2 tablespoons, finely chopped

Balsamic vinegar.....2 teaspoons

Extra virgin olive oil.....4 tablespoons, divided

Black pepper.....1 teaspoon

Cooking spray

Directions

Preheat the oven to 400 degrees. Prepare a baking sheet with cooking spray and set aside.

Pour two tablespoons of olive oil on the cod. Work the oil into the meat then season with pepper.

Roast until the cod is tender and cooked through, about fifteen minutes.

Heat the remaining two tablespoons of oil in a pan over low heat. Add shallot and cook until soft. Add the cherry tomatoes and cook until they begin to soften. Add the capers, olives, vinegar and oregano. Stir for about half a minute.

Plate the cod and spoon the warm tapenade over the cod.

Serve with sautéed kale or spinach and quinoa or orzo.

Butternut Squash Pilaf

Serves 8

Ingredients

Butternut squash.....2 pounds peeled, halved and seeded

Extra virgin olive oil.....1 tablespoon

Red onion.....1 finely chopped

Garlic clove.....1 minced

Water.....2 tablespoons

Tomato paste.....1 tablespoon

Brown rice.....1 cup parboiled

Vegetable broth.....1 - 14 ounce can of vegetable broth

White wine.....1/2 cup

Fennel fronds.....1/2 cup, chopped

Oregano.....2 tablespoons, chopped

Cinnamon.....dash

Black pepper.....to taste

Salt.....1/2 teaspoon

Directions

Grate the butternut squash through the large holes of a box grater.

In a cast iron skillet heat the olive oil on medium heat. Add the red onion and garlic clove. Stir. Allow the onion to turn opaque, about ten minutes.

In a small bowl add two tablespoons of water and the tomato paste. Mix together and transfer to the skillet of onions and garlic. Add parboiled brown rice and stir to coat.

Slowly add the butternut squash to the skillet and allow the squash to reduce down. After it has reduced down increase the heat to medium high and add the broth and wine to the skillet. Cover and bring to a boil.

Reduce the heat to medium low and cook covered until the rice has absorbed most of the liquid and the squash is tender, about twenty minutes.

Add fennel fronds, oregano, cinnamon, salt and pepper. Gently stir to mix. Remove from heat and let stand for five minutes before serving.

Mediterranean Kale

Serves 6

Ingredients

Kale.....12 cups, chopped

Lemon.....1 - 2 tablespoons lemon juice

Extra virgin olive oil.....1 tablespoon or as needed

Garlic.....1 tablespoon, minced

Soy sauce.....1 teaspoon

Salt.....1/4 teaspoon

Black pepper.....to taste

Directions

Using a steamer, fill the lower half of the pan with water and place on high heat.

Bring the water to a boil.

In a strainer, clean and rinse the kale then place it in the top part of the steamer

Insert the basket of kale into the steamer and place the lid on top for five minutes.

In a medium bowl, add olive oil, soy sauce, lemon juice, minced garlic, salt and black pepper.

Whisk the ingredients together then add the steamed kale. Stir to blend. Serve.

Spinach and Feta Pita Bake with Mushrooms and Tomatoes

Serves 6

Ingredients

Sun-dried tomato pesto.....6 ounces

Whole wheat pita bread.....6 - 6 inch

Roma tomatoes.....2 chopped

Fresh spinach.....1 bunch, rinsed and chopped

Mushrooms.....4 sliced

Feta cheese.....1/2 cup

Parmesan cheese.....2 tablespoons, grated

Extra-virgin olive oil.....3 tablespoons

Black pepper.....to taste

Directions

Preheat the oven to 350 degrees.

On a large baking sheet, place the whole wheat pita bread in rows and spread the top of each pita with the tomato pesto.

Add the Roma tomatoes, mushrooms, spinach, feta cheese and parmesan cheese.

Sprinkle the extra-virgin olive oil over the top and add black pepper to taste.

Bake in the oven until the bread is crispy, about twelve minutes.

Remove from the oven and cut into four quarters then transfer to a platter. Serve.

Greek Tzatziki

Makes 5 cups

Ingredients

Plain Greek strained yogurt - 32 ounces

English cucumber.....1/2 with peel, grated (box grater only)

Garlic clove.....1 pressed

Lemon.....1-2 tablespoons lemon juice and 1-2 teaspoons lemon zest, grated

Extra-virgin olive oil.....2 tablespoons

Fresh dill.....3 tablespoons, chopped

Black pepper..... 1 tablespoon

Sea salt.....1 tablespoon, divided

Directions

Grate the cucumber and transfer it to a small bowl. Add half a tablespoon of salt. Stir together then let it sit so that the liquid accumulates on the bottom.

Note: Do not use an automatic food processor. Use the hand held box grater for best results.

In a medium bowl, add the Greek strained yogurt. It will be thicker than standard Greek yogurt. Add the garlic, olive oil, lemon zest, dill, pepper and half a tablespoon of salt then whisk the ingredients together.

Next, return to the bowl of cucumber. Strain the juice from the cucumbers and pat them dry with a paper towel.

Add the strained cucumber to the yogurt mixture and combine. Transfer to a serving dish. Best if chilled before serving.

Roasted Red Pepper Dip

Makes 1 ¾ cups

Ingredients

Feta cheese.....8 ounces feta cheese

Red bell peppers.....2 roasted

Garlic clove.....1 minced

Plain Greek yogurt.....1/4 cup

Cayenne pepper.....to taste

Directions

Roasted Bell Peppers:

Preheat the oven to a low broil and place the rack six to eight inches from the heat source.

Place the bell peppers on a baking sheet then place the baking sheet on the appropriate oven rack keeping the oven door ajar. Watch the peppers as they toast.

After a few minutes, pull the rack out and turn the peppers with a pair of tongs then return them to the oven and toast.

Continue this process until the peppers are nice and toasty all around. This should take five to ten minutes for the whole process. When toasted, remove them from the baking sheet and set aside to cool. Turn the oven off.

Feta and Red Pepper Mix:

In a blender, add the feta cheese, garlic and yogurt. Pulse the blender a couple times to mix. Return to the roasted peppers and cut them into strips. Add the peppers to the blender.

Pulse the blender several times to ensure an even mixture of ingredients. Add cayenne pepper to taste.

Strawberries with Minted Yogurt

Serves 4

Ingredients

Plain Greek yogurt.....1/2 cup

Buttermilk.....1/2 cup

Fresh mint.....1 ½ teaspoons, chopped

Vanilla extract......1/8 teaspoon

Strawberries.....3 cups, sliced

Sugar.....1 tablespoon

Directions

In a medium bowl, add yogurt, buttermilk, mint, sugar and vanilla. Whisk the ingredients together until creamy smooth.

Slice the strawberries into four glass jars and spoon the minty yogurt over the strawberries. Sit some strawberries up in the yogurt to top. Serve immediately.

Baby Tiramisu

Serves 6

Ingredients

Nonfat ricotta cheese.....1/2 cup

Confectioner's sugar.....2 tablespoons

Vanilla extract.....1/2 teaspoon

Ground cinnamon.....1/8 teaspoon

Ladyfingers..... 12

Brewed espresso or strong coffee.....4 tablespoons, divided

Bittersweet chocolate chips.....2 tablespoons, melted

Directions

In a large bowl, combine the ricotta cheese, sugar, vanilla extract, and cinnamon. In a 9 x 5 inch pan place six ladyfingers on the bottom. Drizzle two tablespoons of espresso or strong coffee over the ladyfingers. Add a layer of ricotta cheese then add another layer of the ladyfingers. Drizzle the last of the coffee and melted chocolate on top. Refrigerate for twenty minutes until chocolate sets.

Frosted Almond Date Shake

Serves 4

Ingredients

Fresh dates.....1/3 cup, pitted and chopped

Water....2 tablespoons warm

Vanilla almond milk.....2 cups, chilled

Plain Greek yogurt.....1/2 cup

Banana.....1 very ripe, frozen

Ice cubes.....4

Ground nutmeg.....1/8 teaspoon plus extra for garnish

Directions

In a small bowl add the chopped dates and sprinkle with the warm water. Let soak for five minutes to soften and then drain or pat dry with a paper towel. In a blender, combine the yogurt, almond milk, banana, dates, ice cubes and one eighth teaspoon of nutmeg. Blend until smooth and frothy, about thirty seconds.

Pour into tall, chilled glasses and garnish each with a dusting of nutmeg.

Conclusion

Congratulations on finishing the book! I truly enjoyed writing this book and sharing as much information as I thought was necessary in order for you to understand and apply the Mediterranean diet to your life.

I hope that you feel equipped and ready to dive into Mediterranean style eating and do whatever it takes to achieve optimal health and vitality!

Can I ask you a favor?

If you received value from this book I'd like to ask you a small favor? In order for me to help as many people as possible experience the amazing benefits of the Mediterranean diet I need your help.

If you could take a moment and post a positive review of this book on Amazon that would help others find the book more easily and allow them to begin benefiting from it.

My passion is to help people transform their health and their lives by sharing what I've learned about dieting and weight loss, so thank you in advance for helping me out in this way. I really appreciate it!

Other books by Gina Crawford

Mediterranean Diet Cookbook

DASH Diet for Beginners

DASH Diet Recipes

Sugar Detox for Beginners

Sugar Free Recipes

Paleo for Beginners

5:2 Diet for Beginners

5:2 Diet Recipes

Available on Amazon

About the Author

"Getting healthy, achieving your goal weight, and loving life is only a read away!"

Hi, I'm Gina and I'm a health and "all things natural" enthusiast, author, mother, and wife.

Years ago I was overweight, exhausted, unhappy, and desperately aching for a better life. One day, gruelingly tired of my situation, I started researching everything I could on health, weight loss, and transforming my life. I often felt overwhelmed by the amount of information I was trying to absorb and the changes I had to make, but I persevered and eventually managed to turn my life around one book and one bite at a time.

Now I'm determined to share what I've learned in a direct, straight to the point kind of way that will allow others to achieve maximum results in a short amount of time.

I'm passionate about every book I write and my goal with each book is to make it simple and concise, yet power-packed with the necessary information you need to transform your life.

I have learned first-hand the incredible value of healing ourselves with natural organic foods, natural remedies, exercise, and a positive mindset.

When I'm not writing, I love spending time with my family, cooking, walking, biking, and reading.

My hope is that my books will help you live a healthier, better, more passionate, alive life!

Printed in Great Britain
by Amazon